CHOICE OF HABIT

"In walking by a mirror fast
I vaguely wondered whom I passed;
I backed up several steps to see,
and what a shock!
That 'shock' was me."

Reader's Digest, January 1970

CHOICE
of
HABIT

Poise, Free Movement and the
Practical Use of the Body

by

JACK VINTEN FENTON
D.L.C., D.P.A., Dip. Soc. Studies

Headmaster, de Stafford County Secondary School, Caterham.
Former Headmaster, Woodhatch Primary School, Reigate.
Former Senior Lecturer in Physical and Health Education,
Wandsworth Training College for Teachers, London.

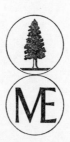

MACDONALD & EVANS LTD
8 John Street, London, WC1N 2HY
1973

First published March 1973

MACDONALD AND EVANS LIMITED

1973

ISBN : 0 7121 0335 X

Printed in Great Britain by
UNWIN BROTHERS LIMITED
OLD WOKING, SURREY

Foreword

Ten years ago I was just one of countless habitual sufferers from what is commonly known as "slipped discs." Then a "good fairy" in the disguise of the director of my then current production suggested that I might benefit from what I now affectionately call The Alexander Method of conscious corrective control of the body.

At the risk of sounding rather fulsome, I can honestly say that since my very first lesson a whole new life has been made possible for me. For the first time I was not relying solely on outside influences to correct the damage to my poorly used body, but I actually did have a "Choice of Habit."

During the past ten years it has proved to be an ever-widening source of investigation, discovery, increased awareness and strength. Indeed, I can think of nothing more wonderful than to be able to pass on this gift to my children, their children and their children's children.

Please allow me to commend to you this book by Mr. Jack Fenton by quoting Professor John Dewey:

"But the method [outlined in this book] is not one of remedy; it is one of constructive education. Its proper field of application is with the young, with the growing generation, in order that they may come to possess as early as possible in life a correct standard of sensory appreciation and self-judgement. When once a reasonably adequate part of a new generation has become properly co-ordinated, we shall have assurance for the first time that men and women in the future will be able to stand on their own feet, equipped with satisfactory psycho-physical equilibrium, to meet with readiness, confidence and happiness instead of with fear, confusion and discontent, the buffetings and contingencies of their surroundings."

NYREE DAWN PORTER

Preface

Modern life can make considerable demands on all of us and especially upon the nervous energy of most men, women and children. This book is an attempt to show how the wear and tear on our bodies can be alleviated and prevented. It shows how many of our habitual movements bring on unnecessary tiredness, reduce our occupational efficiency, and can even produce painful conditions and complaints, often accepted as the penalties of growing old.

A lucky few may naturally have good movement and management of their bodies, but for most of us the skills of good use and sound body mechanics are not spontaneous, they have to be taught. Informal chats with children, even at the age of five or six, reveal that they experience aches and pains in the feet, hips, back and neck.

It is logical that teaching good use should begin as early in life as possible. Experience and experiments have shown that a *preventative* scheme in schools, before habits become set, would avoid much suffering and wasted time for millions of individuals and, incidentally, save the nation the vast expense of production time lost because workers are absent through occupational strain and injury. An *awareness* of the factors involved in acquiring and maintaining good use of the body can do nothing but good.

The suggestions put forward in this book should be of help and interest to parents and all concerned with young people, teachers, lecturers in colleges of education and further education and youth leaders; all ages should benefit from reading it.

The book is copiously illustrated with line drawings and photographs, and it is recognised that the quality of some of the latter may leave something to be desired. However, it was considered important that the actual photography should not make the children self-conscious, so special lighting was not used and the camera was placed as unobtrusively as possible. It was felt that what the illustrations finally chosen had to say about the way we move far outweighed any imperfections. A list of common postural and anatomical terms is given in the Glossary.

Acknowledgments

Grateful acknowledgment is made to the many people without whose help and continual encouragement this book would never have been written.

Thanks are due to the specialist Alexander teachers, in particular to Mr. Donald Grant, M.A., whose infectious enthusiasm was largely responsible for the success of the six-month primary school project described in this book, and to Mrs. Joyce Benson for similar work on the secondary school project; to Dr. Wilfred Barlow, M.A., B.M., B.Ch., who has allowed a number of his cases of postural re-education to be mentioned, and to Mr. Roland Earl, Senior Inspector of Schools to the London Borough of Sutton and former Inspector of Primary Education to the Surrey Education Committee, who gave such great assistance with the preparation of the script.

The help is much appreciated too, of the many teachers in schools and establishments of further education, youth leaders and firms' Education Officers throughout the country, who completed the questionnaires and the head teachers and principals who made the necessary facilities available.

January 1973

J. V. FENTON

Contents

List of Illustrations

CHAPTER I

What Causes Bad Habit?

Introduction

For some years now, an attempt has been made to develop a scientific approach to health that would help to counteract the considerable demands that modern life makes upon the nervous energy of most men and women. This book is an attempt to show how this wear and tear on our bodies can be alleviated and prevented. It shows how many of our habitual movements create unnecessary tiredness and reduce our occupational and industrial efficiency. It describes how teachers can help boys and girls to improve their performance in games and sports and everyday activities by good management of the body.

The need for such a book became apparent when the author was developing a scheme of physical education to satisfy the interests of young people between the ages of fifteen and eighteen which at the same time would help to remedy some of the faults in their posture which were obvious from observations. Research findings underlined this need.

For example, an analysis of the occupational activities performed by a sample of 1,200 boys at work brought to light certain weaknesses, as did an analysis of the daily activities performed by children and young people between five and eighteen years of age at school. The results of both showed very clearly that to manage ourselves and our bodies well, all of us, not only young people, do need to give them a little thought and a little care.

Nobody expects an appliance or instrument to function perfectly with no thought, no maintenance and no care. It seems logical to treat the human body in the same way. Unfortunately, all of us do not naturally make good use of our bodies—we often make uneconomical use of ourselves and need to be taught how to improve. Research findings indicate that the earlier this takes place in a child's life, before set habits are formed, the better.

It must be stressed first of all that the reader of this book will not be in a position to correct some physical defect or faulty habit of use merely by reading its suggestions. The tennis player or the cricketer does not improve a stroke by reading about it. Words and instructions can only have meaning when accompanied by the sensory experience attached to them; children literally cannot do many things they are told through lack of previous physical experience.

A lucky few may have naturally good posture and movement, but there are many children today who suffer from poor posture, un-co-ordinated movement and undue tension. Although many national health habits have changed for the good, our use of our bodies has not improved (see Plates 14 and 15).

Formation of Bad Habits

One of the main obstacles to making the most efficient use of the body is that until children learn how to direct their attention properly they have little or no idea how they move. They know that they stand, sit, and walk, but they have very little idea how they do these things. They do what they feel to be right, though very often this can be shown to be fundamentally unsound.

Consider, for example, the way that some children sit when they are writing; weight unevenly distributed, body hunched, neck stiff, brows knitted, eyes strained and their pens gripped with excessive tension. Of course, they feel that it is perfectly natural, and they are usually unaware of the strain, although they may wonder, later on, why they have headaches, discomfort in the neck, shoulder and wrist, and perhaps feel unduly tired.

In teaching children to write, these faults should not be allowed to arise, for it is certain that most faulty habits of movement and posture are formed in childhood. Unfortunately, the teacher is so anxious to get the child to write that she spends little time in helping him to maintain a good position while he is doing so.

How, then, can children learn to use their bodies so that they serve them better, last longer, and actually look and feel at ease?

A simple instance of how what is habitual "feels" right may be seen if a pupil who always stands with rather tightly braced shoulders and pulled-in chin is asked to stand easily erect looking ahead. He will do so according to custom and assume that he has complied. When the teacher indicates the way this can be effected by releasing all the effort not needed for standing erect, the pupil feels slouched, round-shouldered and slovenly, even when to an observer he is, in fact, erect, rightly aligned and alert.

Another example of this habitual feeling was observed during a dancing lesson when eight-year-old David, who normally leans forward, was asked to stand up a little straighter. On being given a better alignment by his teacher as the verbal instruction was of little avail, he cried "Oh, Miss, don't let go. I'm falling backwards!"

Through a knowledge of simple anatomy, children can be shown how their bodies are constructed and how they work. Many children (and adults for that matter) think the joint by which they lean forward is much higher than it really is, and they literally bend their backs when they should be moving from their hip joints. This sensory appreciation of exactly where the head balances on the top of the vertebral column— it is roughly between the ears—can prevent many a headache.

By this postural approach to physical education, many children can be helped towards more effective action, as can the ordinary adult who wishes to be fitter.

Bad habits are all too often acquired in childhood if an action is repeatedly performed in the wrong way, and no correction is given. A child may imitate the bad habit of an adult. We may become tense through anxiety, and both illness and injury can cause poor posture or movement. We try to develop sound habits of speech, cleanliness, punctuality and so on in our children. But habits which may affect the whole future well-being of a child, even deforming the framework of his body or causing pain, seldom get the same correction. One reason is because many parents and teachers fail to recognise such faults, even when they see them.

The skills of good use and sound body mechanics are rarely inherited as a natural gift, they have to be taught just as the skills of reading and numeracy have to be taught. Speaking generally, the pre-school child does have sound body use (*see* Plate 2), but it can be readily observed that many habits are well established and conditioned by the time the child arrives at school when he is five years old. Often the particular mannerisms of mother or father walking—the tilt of the head or carriage of the trunk—are mirrored in the child. The gentle suggestion of the reception class teacher that the children should line up smartly at the door immediately brings to Tommy's body the stiffness of the guard on parade. With tense hollow back, locked elbows, straight fingers and head held up he puts into operation his best standing position, as envisaged from some pre-school experience (*see* Plate 10).

Even at the age of five or six, informal chats reveal that children experience aches and pains in their feet, hips, back and neck, while observation shows clearly the related poor use of their bodies (*see* Plates 3, 5, 6 and 7). Many of the children's normal movements show poor mechanical use of the trunk and limbs, which should have been noticed and improved from the beginning.

Mummy does not hesitate to correct Mary when she speaks badly, because she knows that bad speech soon becomes a habit. But she rarely corrects Mary when she performs some physical action badly, simply because very few mothers (or fathers) are aware of the soundest and safest ways of using the body. Neither are they aware of the many completely unnecessary movements which are made and which cause unnecessary tiredness.

Nor—until Mary complains of a pain—are many mothers and fathers aware of the movements which children make which may cause them harm. Quite often there are no readily observable symptoms, so that abnormalities go unnoticed until they become gross.

It is not suggested, however, that children's activities should be limited in any way, only that every child needs help in the very early years in learning how to use its body well. Mothers and fathers can do a great deal by encouraging lots of the right kind of movement. But the great majority of children cannot "pick up" sound physical habits without assistance, any more than they can "pick up" reading and writing without help and guidance. They are surrounded by influences from which they can develop right or wrong habits or attitudes without the ability, because of their lack of experience, to choose the most satisfactory for themselves.

Children should be lithe and agile, with easy-flowing movement; they should look good and attractive in action. Yet when many five-year-olds start school they are stiff, tense and awkward in action. Lots of them need as much help with physical skills as they do with academic skills, yet *they are literally taught to run before they can walk*. Ankle, knee and hip joints seldom perform their allotted tasks in walking and it is no exaggeration to say that many parents and teachers are quite unaware of the potential movements of these joints.

The five-year-old has already developed some quite firm habits by the time he sets foot in school. On that very first morning are not teachers rather too eager to get something into their hands, be it crayon, chalk, brush, learner's pencil or plasticine, instead of letting them "feel" their way about the room, experiencing their surroundings and observing where things are? Are teachers perhaps so keen to get something done that they do not pay enough attention to how it is being done? Does Willie have to grip his new crayon in a vice-like grip and with knuckles showing white (*see* Plate 11)? Does he have to make marks into several layers of the pad while sitting on his foot on the seat of the chair?

It is not being suggested that he should sit up straight in his chair and "draw like teacher," because he cannot. Let him sit on his foot if he wants to. Let him kneel or squat or even lie on the floor, but let him do so in an easy and free manner, devoid of unnecessary tension. Let him experiment with his hand, holding his crayon *tightly* while trying to put something on the paper, and then show him how to hold it *lightly* and easily—and notice the difference (*see* Plate 11). In short, teachers should pay attention first of all to the way things are done, and secondly to what is done. And they should do so right from the start, from the first day in the reception class.

Watch a child writing a composition, his body twisted to the right, one shoulder drooping below the other. There is the beginning of lateral curvature of the spine, for "such a position adopted, without correction, day after day, becomes such a habit that even when the child is in an erect position he holds himself like that."

Many children disabled through injury can be made more comfortable, mentally and physically, by being taught to use even a damaged body more effectively. A boy of eleven in a primary school in which this approach was used suffered from the after-effects of polio. With one leg in irons and all movement carried out on crutches, he found that he could move with much less discomfort, at football, for instance, when he could move with considerable speed, by practising the principles taught him.

Learning to "Stop"

Children will naturally be more tense than usual during their first few days at school for it is bound to be a slightly anxious time for them. Teachers, therefore, should make sure that the environment savours of freedom, not only in the activities they can do, but in the way they are encouraged to do them. They should be allowed to "ease off" physically— not, that is, easing off in the usual sense of doing less work, but a muscular easing off. They should be encouraged to relax. This does not mean that any kind of vigorous work is to be avoided—vigorous activities can be performed in a released, smooth way, or they can be done in a tense, strained and constricted way. The teacher's job is to encourage the first way, for as already indicated the great majority of children do not perform well naturally.

Through individual instruction and group work boys and girls can be shown the right and wrong way to perform simple bodily movements. They can be encouraged to have a moment of "stop"—the ability to come to rest before the jump, the climb, the vault or whatever activity it might be.

They can be taught how to come to the edge of the high box in preparation for a downward jump (as a diver approaches the diving board) and go through, momentarily, this simple procedure: feel how the box holds them up, that is consciously

PLATES I (*a*) AND I (*b*)

LET THE SPINE LENGTHEN
Develop an expanded posture

PLATE I (*a*)—RIGHT

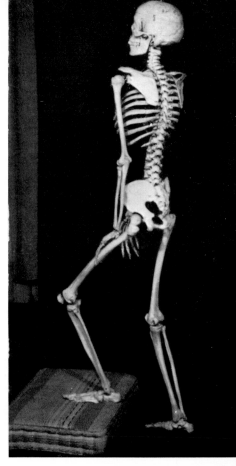

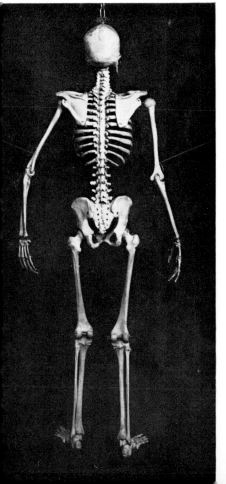

PLATE I (*b*)—LEFT

ALLOW *the joints to ease*
AVOID *pulling-in of joint surfaces*

PLATE 2—RIGHT
*Most infants move
in a graceful,
co-ordinated
way*

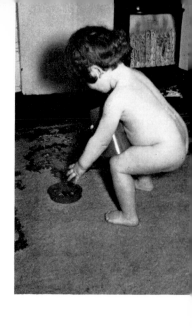

PLATE 3—BELOW
*By the age of five
and six years, posture
has all too often
seriously deteriorated*

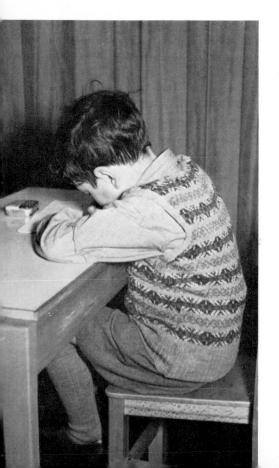

PLATE 4—BELOW
*Postural improvement
can only be achieved
by special
instruction*

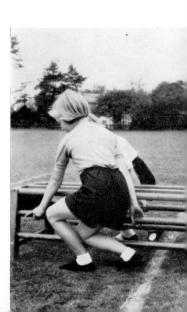

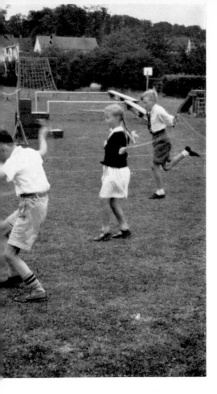

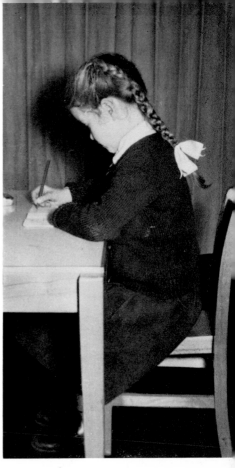

PLATE 5
*Girl skipping with good use,
boys skipping with poor use*

PLATE 6
Same girl sitting with good use

Our HABITUAL POSTURE *is carried into whatever activity is performed*

PLATE 7
*Same boys
lifting with
poor use*

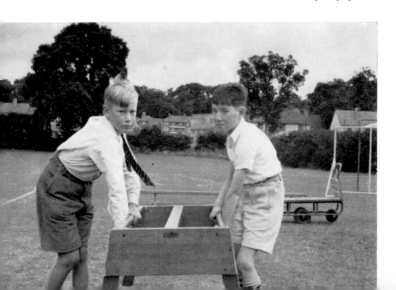

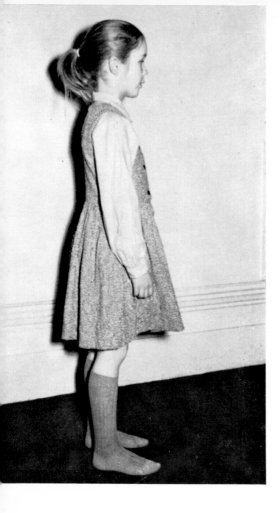

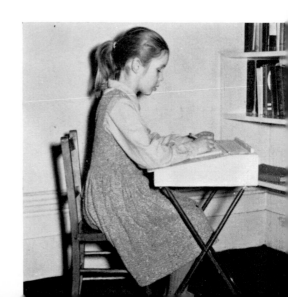

PLATES 8 and 9
*Girl showing good use
in standing and
sitting*

PLATE 8

PLATE 9

to experience support; look ahead without staring or "looking through" things; let the whole body ease upwards, "grow" as it were; feel their head lightly balanced, shoulders resting lightly; finally, decide what they are going to do.

This ability to "collect themselves," or "check-over" and form a clear intention of what to do next can lead to a considerable improvement in their posture and movement. It was most noticeable during television film of the 1972 Olympic Games events that competitors carried out the fundamentals of this technique to attain their optimum performance. First they could be seen making every effort to relax, and second forming a clear intention of what they were aiming at. The high jumper, for example, had a long pause whilst paying attention to the height of the bar. (One would normally think of "concentrating" on the bar, but the word concentration conjures up a furrowing of the brows, etc., and therefore tension.) This was paying attention without unnecessary tension.

It is only when these two points are accomplished that the best performance can be achieved, whether it be at sport, at work or study. It is an ability which grows with practice, and when it comes it is possible for the teacher and children to correct faulty habits of movement and body mechanics. For example, the child who on rising from a chair pulls his head back on his spine, lifting himself, as it seems, by his shoulders, will persist in this uneconomic habit until he acquires some ability "to check-over."

The reason for this is that when he is told by his teacher to stand, his body responds willy-nilly, in his habitual and harmful way. What he has to do is to learn to use his body so that he can disperse the activity irrelevant to the job of standing up. Momentarily, he must come to rest and allow himself a choice of how he will stand up. He may choose to direct his head forward and lengthen his back before straightening his legs as the weight of his body comes over his feet. This gets him up, but it is not what "standing" meant to him before, for he had to refuse his immediate response to his teacher's direction and *choose* to respond quite differently. With practice, the new and more efficient response becomes automatic.

It is very important to recognise that the whole crux of this

B

approach is based on the principle that *the thought of an action is sufficient to ennervate the muscles which habitually perform it.* The mere thought of standing, just described, prepared the muscles which habitually help us in this movement. If the movement is faulty, we must, as it were, wipe the slate of habit clean, start afresh, choose and develop a new improved pattern.

The use of this moment of refusal or stop as distinct from a sudden stiffening by "applying the brakes" is a principle of considerable importance in physical education, and it has been used to help children who were having difficulty with reading and arithmetic as well as in movement and activity. Curiously enough, American educationists who have been greatly influenced by Professor Dewey's advocacy of "learning through doing" have not taken equally close account of his insistence that postural education must be the basis if such learning is to be effective.

The obvious and logical time to start paying as much attention to these physical skills as is paid to other educational skills is in the primary school, and teachers should continue to encourage and develop them throughout the child's school life.

Adult Habit and Attendant Disorders

How many adults suffer needlessly from sciatica or the more fashionable "slipped disc" because of their own faulty lifting habits? Sixty-six per cent of children tested in school show that they do not know how to lift safely, whilst a senior army officer has related how during the second World War hospital wards contained many soldiers suffering from hernia because they had lifted shell cases in an unsound manner. How many older industrial workers carry the unnecessary stigma of round shoulders through bending over their machines all day? How many housewives get back-ache through bad standing habits and how many office workers quite literally have a "pain in the neck" because they fail to sit correctly? Book-keepers, typists, proof readers, dress-makers, and school teachers with lots of marking to do are especially prone to such pains. Indeed, anyone who is forced to hold his head rigidly in a particular position is likely to get a headache.

Yet the *cause* of the pain can be removed, not by heat and massage, which are merely temporary palliatives, but by teaching the man, woman or child to perform whatever activity they have to do in the most efficient manner and without undue muscular tension.

How many people "whose feet are killing them" realise the important part they play in the general health and efficiency of the body because they are directly concerned with posture? Countless foot ailments are found among shop assistants and factory workers because they are most apt to throw themselves off-balance and once corns and bunions are formed they become aggravated because the sufferers try to find relief by the same means—an off-balance stance.

Loss of time, slower work, irritation and inefficiency are a direct result of aching feet. Workmen like house-painters and plasterers who stand for a long time on the rungs of a ladder can develop neuralgia of the foot; delivery drivers who habitually jump from their vehicles develop a painful enlargement of the first ball joint, and men and women who spend a great deal of time driving cars and lorries suffer from a type of callus known as "chauffeur's foot." Yet nearly all these adults' foot troubles could be checked in childhood by paying far more attention to suppleness, sound muscles and good tone, which are the essentials of healthy feet.

There are many other disorders in addition to brachial neuritis, pain in the back and in the joints, and "slipped disc," which are often attributed to or aggravated by mismanagement of the body. There are also the pyschosomatic disorders and those caused by over-tension and anxiety, such as asthma and certain kinds of headaches and indigestion.

Even physical training specialists, unless they are trained in "postural awareness," are not immune from habit-formed defects. For example, a young woman javelin thrower found her repeated twisting movement led to an habitual lateral curvature of the spine, even when she was at rest; a right-handed thrower, too, found that her pain-giving rotary twist of the spine remained with her at rest; the head retraction of the sprinter when at rest, accustomed to breasting the tape desperately, is another typical example.

Conclusions

Bad posture and badly co-ordinated movements are the result of long-standing, unsatisfactory and unconscious responses to the desire to move, stand, sit, walk, lift, and so on. The pupil, therefore, must learn to respond to these everyday impulses in a new way if he is to improve. Mere exercising will not do the trick.

Right from the start parents and teachers should realise why attention to posture is so important, for it is the basis upon which habits of co-ordinated movement can be built, and since really good posture is rarely spontaneous it has to be developed.

Poor posture is often associated with anxiety and nervous tension which show themselves quite early in school life, and it contributes to functional disorders like flat feet, headaches, digestive upsets, asthma and stammering

In suggesting to children how they can become more aware of how their bodies work teachers should advise them to relax where they can and tense only when they have to. It has already been shown that the ability to relax is developed by practice, and boys and girls must develop the ability to detect which muscle groups are tense. They have to learn to save energy by minimising all unnecessary actions and directing essential ones skilfully.

Because it takes time to relax they must be given time to do so, and as they practise the exercises outlined throughout this book, the teacher by observation can discover tense and released muscles and so know when to give the next instruction.

Research into Posture

The Author's Research Projects

Before proceeding to outline ways in which teachers and parents can help their children and themselves use their bodies more effectively it is interesting to note the results of an investigation carried out by the author concerning the daily activities peformed by children and young people at school aged between five and eighteen years. This covered a sample of about one thousand children from schools throughout England and Wales. The aim of this questionnaire (*see* Figs. 1 and 2) was to see what proportion of the various age groups between five and eighteen naturally and habitually chose the most economical position and method of use, for posture is a habit, and whatever posture a child has is carried into whatever activity he performs. The explanatory notes given to teachers were as follows:

This questionnaire is an attempt to determine the main ways by which children of different age groups (five to eighteen years) perform some of their daily activities.

Please enter the total number in the class being checked and the age of the class (years only) as it was at the beginning of the educational year on 1st September last, and use a separate sheet for each age. The marking of each section should be done in the space below it.

To acquire an accurate picture of the present situation, it is necessary that the sheet is completed with the children *unposed*. They may be aware that you are checking something from the sheet in your hand but they will not know what it is. The *habitual pattern* of the child is wanted, and not one that can be approximately attained and held for a few minutes if desired.

Variations of an activity may be seen, other than those shown on any one line. If these variations do not fall into

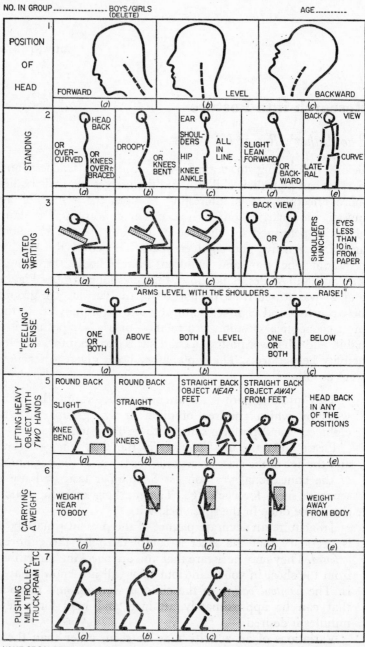

FIG. I—*The questionnaire on children's movement.*

one of the categories given, please enter the number at the beginning of the line.

It is appreciated that children alter their positions (*e.g.* sitting) many times in a short lesson. Thus when checking the "seated writing" line, it is suggested that the check is taken during the first few minutes after the children have started writing.

In many people the kinaesthetic sense is faulty or poorly developed. The line headed "feeling" sense, which should be carried out with closed eyes, is to find out how many children have an accurate interpretation (without looking) of the "arms sideways position."

The lifting and carrying positions might be checked by preparing a group for an obstacle or relay competition, so that four or six children walk to an object (no race), lift it with *two* hands, and then carry it on to a given mark and place it down.

It takes longer to observe the pushing position, so if only one group of the class picked at random, could be checked, it would be much appreciated. The weight of the object lifted, carried or pushed should suit the age of the child and demand normal effort.

None of the teachers was a specialist teacher of posture and none had been specially trained to discern movements or positions which indicated unnecessary tension or malposture.

This enquiry, which was a general one, revealed the fairly obvious and noticeable positions and movements of boys and girls. It did not show the minute deviations of good and bad use. Indeed, it appears likely that the percentage of boys with good use is lower than the graphs suggest.

For example, Plate 18(*a*) in the centre, shows an activity called "lifting the log" being badly performed and causing consider-able unnecessary strain. Plate 18(*b*) shows the same activity being performed with better body mechanics and with less liability to damage and strain—but still not with good use. Notice that the lifter is on his toes, his head is drawn back, not aligned with his trunk and leading it in the lift, and his body is not sufficiently over the weight he is lifting—all of which causes overwork and strain. Yet this boy would have been placed in the best

POSITION OF HEAD	5 No.	5 %	6 No.	6 %	7 No.	7 %	8 No.	8 %	9 No.	9 %	10 No.	10 %	11 No.	11 %	12 No.	12 %	13 No.	13 %	14 No.	14 %	15 No.	15 %	16 No.	16 %	17 No.	17 %	18 No.	18 %	19 No.	19 %
1(a)	20	26	22	18	20	41	7	14	4	5	16	18	37	27	13	23	22	36	13	15	22	31	33	31	11	23	16	36	256	24
(b)	49	64	71	60	25	51	41	84	68	92	63	70	75	54	42	74	32	52	69	78	36	51	60	57	32	68	25	55	688	66
(c)	8	14	26	22	4	8	1	2	2	3	11	12	6	4	2	4	7	11	6	7	12	17	12	11	4	9	4	9	105	10
TOTAL	77		119		49		49		74		90		118		57		61		88		70		105		47		45		1049	
STANDING 2(a)	8	14	20	17	6	12	3	6	6	8	8	9	6	4	1	2	5	10	2	2	6	9	9	9	3	6	10	22	93	9
(b)	8	14	15	13	8	16	5	10	3	4	3	3	9	7	11	19	10	20	6	7	12	18	13	12	15	33	6	13	174	17
(c)	43	56	62	51	24	49	41	84	64	86	64	73	80	58	40	70	23	45	64	71	30	35	40	38	22	58	21	46	618	59
(d)	17	22	17	14	9	18	-	-	1	1	13	15	20	15	3	5	11	12	12	13	16	24	38	36	5	11	12	27	174	17
(e)	6	13	6	5	2	4	-	2	-	1	-	1	-	1	2	4	7	14	8	9	4	6	7	7	3	7	4	9	51	5
TOTAL	77		120		49		49		74		88		138		57		51		90		66		105		46		45		1055	
SEATED WRITING 3(a)	22	28	50	42	12	27	12	24	24	32	35	41	51	37	18	32	20	33	40	46	36	39	53	50	14	29	24	53	401	38
(b)	41	53	25	21	20	44	28	57	40	54	41	48	29	21	27	47	22	36	29	33	23	35	31	30	18	38	18	40	372	35
(c)	14	18	16	13	7	15	8	16	9	12	8	9	19	14	11	19	17	28	10	12	13	20	14	13	10	21	2	4	158	15
(d)	18	33	20	17	5	11	7	14	9	12	11	13	12	9	16	16	9	15	16	18	13	20	22	21	11	23	19	42	172	16
(e)	6	13	14	12	4	9	5	10	21	27	6	7	10	7	-	-	14	23	15	17	32	49	33	31	12	25	-	-	176	16
(f)	40	52	19	16	16	35	16	33	29	39	6	6	25	18	10	18	8	13	19	22	15	23	29	21	8	17	-	-	239	23
TOTAL	77		120		45		49		74		85		138		57		61		87		66		105		48		45		1057	

	1	2	3	4	5	6	7	8	9	10	11	12	13	14	15	16	17	18	19	20	21	22	23	24	25	26	27	28	Total	%
"FEELING" SENSE 4(a)	6	8	30	25	13	26	7	14	12	16	13	14	9	7	14	25	21	34	30	34	14	21	34	32	22	41	29	64	254	24
(b)	38	49	38	31	26	53	31	63	51	69	65	72	78	58	39	68	25	41	50	56	35	53	51	49	30	56	15	33	572	54
(c)	33	43	53	44	10	20	11	22	11	15	12	13	28	21	4	7	15	24	9	10	17	26	20	19	2	4	1	2	226	21
	77		121		49		49		74		90		115		57		61		89		66		105		54		45		1052	
LIFTING 5(a)	16	35	26	31	27	53	28	57	22	30	58	64	96	70	45	79	27	55	41	57	21	31	27	28	24	51	22	49	480	49
(b)	-	2	10	12	3	6	15	30	8	11	3	3	9	7	-	-	11	18	18	25	11	17	12	12	7	15	8	18	116	12
(c)	28	61	43	51	16	30	7	14	43	59	26	29	10	7	11	19	15	25	24	33	32	48	49	40	14	30	14	31	332	34
(d)	-	2	5	6	5	10	1	1	-	1	3	3	-	-	-	2	5	8	4	6	2	3	9	9	2	4	2	4	39	4
(e)	-	-	26	31	7	14	1	1	2	3	-	-	3	2	-	-	5	8	-	-	4	6	6	6	4	9	-	-	57	6
	46		84		51		50		73		90		138		57		60		72		66		97		47		45		976	
CARRYING 6(a)	5	11	52	48	14	27	43	88	64	88	40	44	78	57	20	35	19	32	46	52	29	44	52	54	42	91	-	-	505	51
(b)	14	30	37	34	14	27	29	59	9	12	24	27	38	33	3	5	12	20	12	14	21	32	14	15	10	22	7	16	244	25
(c)	19	41	25	23	23	45	10	20	17	23	34	38	12	10	8	14	20	33	7	8	24	37	22	23	10	22	8	18	239	24
(d)	8	17	46	43	14	27	10	20	47	64	32	36	65	57	46	81	28	47	69	79	21	32	57	60	25	54	30	67	498	50
(e)	-	-	18	17	4	8	6	12	9	12	-	-	-	-	-	-	8	13	18	20	1	2	11	11	4	9	-	-	79	8
	46		108		51		49		73		90		115		57		60		88		66		96		46		45		990	
PUSHING 7(a)	15	20	9	19	11	22	11	22	14	19	48	53	17	15	9	16	11	18	23	26	28	41	10	13	9	31	4	9	219	24
(b)	30	40	14	30	16	31	9	18	5	7	10	11	25	22	8	14	19	31	25	28	16	24	11	14	7	24	14	31	209	23
(c)	30	40	24	51	24	47	29	59	54	74	32	36	73	63	40	70	32	51	40	45	22	23	56	73	13	45	27	60	496	54
% TO NEAREST WHOLE No.	75		47		51		49		73		90		115		57		62		88		66		77		29		43		924	

FIG. 2.—Analysis of daily activities performed by children and young people.

category (line (5c) in Fig. 2) by the non-specialist teacher of posture.

In Plate 18(a) again, notice "rocking the dummy." The boy on the left of the picture pushing the "dummy" has his knees flexed and is in fact leaning slightly backwards, whereas the same activity in Plate 18(b) shows a better mechanical position with the whole body, including the head, aligned and going forward with the push.

Similarly in Plate 18(a) "lifting the sack" is performed by the boy with braced knees causing back strain, while in Plate 18(b) on the right, the knees are flexed, relieving the strain.

When the first photograph was taken, attention was being paid mainly to demonstrating the three different activities. When the second photograph was taken, as well as demonstrating three different activities, the emphasis was more on *how* they were being performed, rather than *what* they were doing.

"Although no one position may be entirely incorrect or correct, some are known to be better than others because they result in less strain and fatigue. This factor alone ultimately affects the well-being of the individual."[5]

One diagram on each line of the questionnaire (*see* Fig. 1) indicates the most advantageous mechanical position for that action:

Position of head	(1(b))	"Feeling" sense	(4(b))
Seated writing	(3(b))	Carrying	(6(d))
Lifting	(5(c))	Pushing	(7(c))
	Standing	(2(c))	

The percentage of boys in each age group showing these positions is given as a graph of each position (*see* Fig. 3). The percentage of the *total* sample is also shown in each case. If we consider the percentage of the total sample found to be *not* showing sound body mechanics, the following figures emerged:

Position of head	34
Standing	41
Seated writing	65
Feeling sense	46
Lifting	66
Carrying	50
Pushing	46

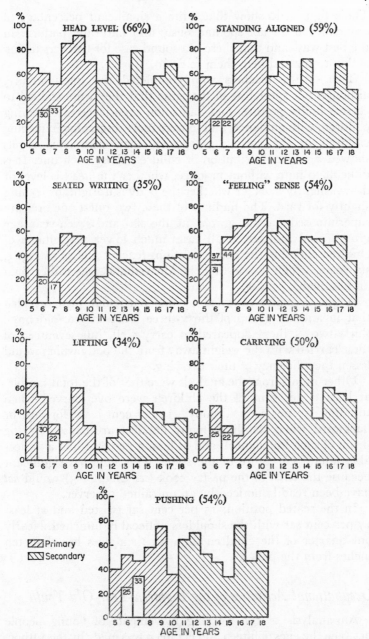

FIG. 3—*Percentage of boys per age group showing* MOST *sound body mechanics.*

These figures do show that quite a significant percentage of our children do not spontaneously and naturally perform in the best way, and that there is a sound case for teachers taking action to try and help them to do so.

Two of the teachers who completed the questionnaire, although not specialists in the sense that they were trained to correct faulty posture, had had some experience of observing children, with guidance, and so were more discerning in placing children in the various categories—their completed sheets showed a wider distribution of children along each line. It is difficult to note without practice, whether the head is level or drawn slightly back, or whether the body is upright, or leaning slightly forward. The findings of these two questionnaires are superimposed on the graphs at the six- and seven-year age groups, and indicate in all cases much lower percentages of children choosing the better positions (except line 4*b* in Fig. 3, six years, which was testing the kinaesthetic *sense* rather than an observable *position*).

A questionnaire returned by one particular firm revealed that in another group of thirty-three fourteen-year-old boys, thirty-two of them appeared to carry well, but seventeen of these carried with the weight away from the body which would lessen the efficiency of their carrying.

Other points from the analysis were that of the total sample, at least 9 per cent of the children were over-curved when standing, 17 per cent "droopy", 17 per cent leant forward or backward when standing (many flat feet are caused by the strain of such imbalance), and at least 5 per cent had a noticeable lateral curvature of the spine. This figure is significant because the twist of the pastry cook (*see* Chapter 3) would *not* have been readily noticed by an untrained observer.

In the seated position, 15 per cent sat twisted and at least 17 per cent sat with the shoulders noticeably hunched. Nearly one-quarter of the children sat with their eyes less than ten inches from the paper.

Occupational Activities of the Eighteen-Year-Old Youth

An analysis of the working movements of young people between the ages of fifteen and eighteen was made by the author, carried out initially as a possible guide in determining the sort of remedial physical education needed for those between fifteen and eighteen years of age at full-time education or at work. It was based on the questionnaire shown in Fig. 4.

At the same time, actual observation of youths forming the National Service intake at eighteen years corroborated many of the findings.

An analysis of the occupational activities performed regularly each day provided valuable material for this book, for there is ample evidence to indicate that occupational movements can produce physical maladjustments. These are discussed in more detail later in the chapter. The facts show that a number of everyday activities are likely to produce round shoulders, whilst the large number of boys who work in the "standing stooped" position each day (58 per cent) is liable to increase this tendency. In fact, the report from the Forces about the National Service men said that the main postural fault found was round shoulders.

Further, as over 81 per cent of these boys stand on their feet most of the day, unless they stand well-aligned and balanced the situation will not be improved. "Standing is the most fatiguing of daily occupations," argued one expert worker in this field in an article in a journal, and another noted that a relatively common postural fault is "shop-girl's hip": shop assistants habitually stand with one knee bent and the opposite buttock pushed out, a position which causes postural back-ache or pain in the abdomen.

The daily activities of any worker, young or old, also include a number of unilateral movements which may produce both pain and some lateral curvature of the spine. The pastry cook mentioned in Chapter 3 is a good example.

Aching and back-ache are often caused by an off-balance stance when standing. Muscle strain, if continued over a period, can have serious effects, not only because of the pain and discomfort that it causes, but because the muscles themselves become chemically injured by the piling up of lactic acid within their tissue. They may eventually become incapable of responding to nervous impulses, they may become over-tense and unable to relax, or they may lose tone and become flabby. In either case, the condition is a serious one, which may take

A Name _____ Date of birth _____ Age _____

B Occupation _____

C District in which you work _____
   Is it rural, small town, suburban, large town?
      (cross out those not applicable)

D How do you usually go to and from work ? _____
   How long does it usually take there and back? _____

E What footwear do you most often wear at work? _____

F Do you take part regularly each week in any physical activities ?
                     e.g. games, P.T. class, etc. _____

G From the following, number two in order (I,2) at which you spend most time, each day at work

   Standing upright _____
   Standing stooped, e.g. over
   bench or desk _____
   Seated _____
   Lying down _____
   Strolling e.g. about the office, etc. _____
   Kneeling _____
   Any other position ? _____

H The following are activities which you may do in your normal daily work
   Indicate in the appropriate column whether the activity is regular, occasional or rare

	Most regular	Occasional	Rare or never
I PUSHING heavy objects			
2 PULLING heavy objects			
3 LIFTING heavy objects (a) off the ground (off bench, etc.)			
4 CARRYING heavy objects (a) with two hands			
(b) with one hand			
(c) on the back			
(d) in front			
(e) on the shoulder			
5 BENDING (a) downwards			
(b) sideways			
(c) backwards			
6 DIGGING, shovelling, etc.			
7 REACHING upward above the head			
8 CLIMBING using legs and hands (e.g. ladder)			
using legs only (e.g. stairs)			
using hands only (e.g. ropes)			
9 SAWING, filing or similar movements			
IO HAMMERING (a) with one hand			
(b) swinging large hammer			
II Use FINGERS (a) both hands			
(b) one hand			
I2 Use WRISTS (a) both hands			
(b) one hand			
I3 CYCLING (how long usually ?) _____			
I4 WALKING (how long usually?) _____			
I5 Any other activity ? _____			

FIG. 4—*The questionnaire on activities performed regularly by boys between fifteen and eighteen years at work.*

time to overcome. If everyday movements were more generally performed correctly much unnecessary fatigue, weariness and often pain would be avoided.

The importance of physical education in helping to prevent the onset of fatigue, rather than merely helping people to recuperate when they have become fatigued, is not always appreciated. Physiological fatigue seems to be so general in character that once a state of fatigue has been produced, rest is the only cure. Correct habits do encourage economy of energy, particularly noticeable as more skill is acquired, and this is clearly an additional method of preventing fatigue.

As well over half of the boys between fifteen and eighteen spend most of their day standing stooped over a bench or a counter and 80 per cent never reach above their head at work, games which make them jump and reach upward should have a special place in their physical education, *e.g.* basket ball, volley ball and netball. (This lack of mobility in the shoulders is also borne out by an observer[4] who stated that of ninety-four ex-grammar school students entering training college in the early 1960s, only fifty-three could raise their arms vertically, a situation which has not changed.

"Actions repeated innumerable times for years on end, such as all our habitual actions, mould even the bones, let alone the muscular envelope. The physical faults that appear in our body long after we were born are mainly the result of activity we have imposed on it. Faulty modes of standing and walking produce flat feet, and it is the mode of standing and walking that must be corrected and not the feet."[5]

1. THE TOTTENHAM INVESTIGATION INTO THE PHYSIQUE OF
   CHILDREN AT THE AGE OF FIFTEEN YEARS

An investigation carried out with school children in Tottenham on behalf of the Research Board for the Correlation of Medical Science and Physical Education (1948) produced some interesting data.

The main findings revealed two significant facts:

(*a*) "Percentages of those with special needs will be seen to increase with age," and (*b*) a "large group of children seemed to be likely to profit by re-education."

Age Group	Total no. of children	Total no. with special physical needs	Percentages with special physical needs
2–5	196	58	29·6
6–9	299	112	37·4
10–13	990	633	67·0
14–17	367	251	68·0
Totals	1,852	1,054	56·9

According to workers in the field of posture, the proportion of children and adults with defects is still higher when the misuse of the body involves unnecessary muscular and nervous tension. These defects are not readily observable visually, but can quickly be discovered tactually.

2. OTHER REPORTS AND ENQUIRIES

The Report of the Chief Medical Officer of the Ministry of Education for the years 1946–47 noted "a significant change in physical education with a view to replacing unnecessary tenseness during exercise by ease of movement." It also mentioned that during this period there was "an extension of remedial work where special exercises were introduced to correct postural defects. Reports show that though far-reaching improvements are now being introduced into the general schemes of physical activity in schools, the proportion of children requiring treatment is high."

Another Report presented by the Parliamentary Secretary to the Ministry of Education at a conference organised by the Central Council of Health Education and quoted in *The Times Educational Supplement*, stated that "as many as 60 per cent of children in primary schools were suffering from a slight physical defect."

A Divisional Education Medical Officer in the Home Counties wrote in his annual report that "minor crippling and postural deformities represented about one-fourth of the total defects

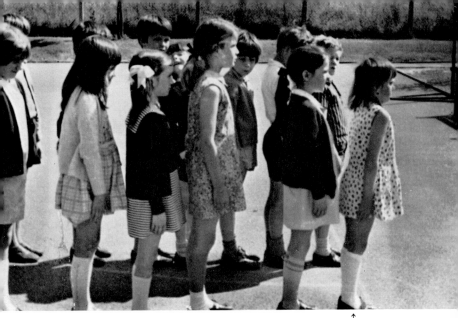

PLATE 10(a)

PLATES 10(a) AND 10(b)

*Children standing; note that those arrowed are
over-tense throughout the body*

PLATE 10(b)

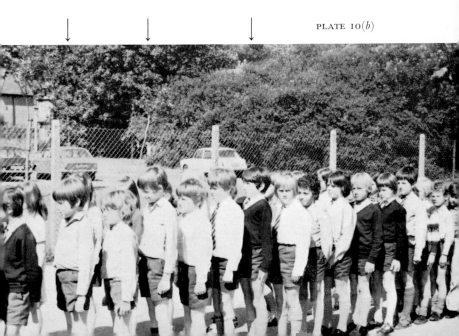

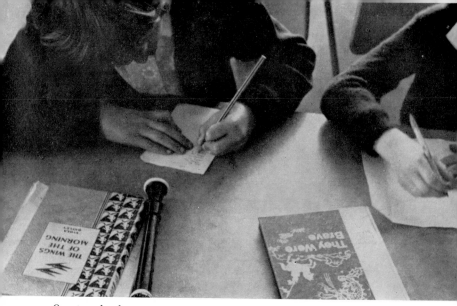

Over-tense hand   *Better use*

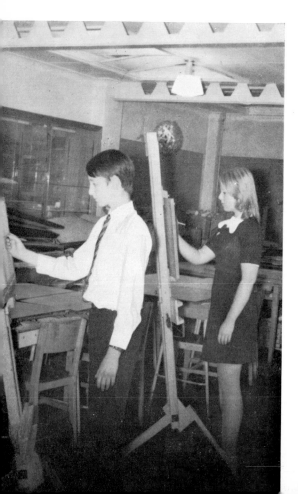

PLATE 11—ABOVE
Children writing

PLATE 12—LEFT
*Painting, showing good
use, though shadow on
boy's neck shows tension*

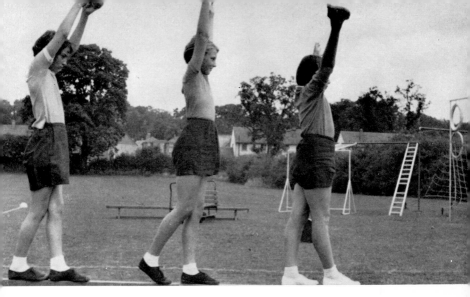

Poor use—limited shoulder movement

Good use—fullest possible use made of joints

Poor use—limited shoulder movement

PLATE 13(a)—ABOVE
Raising arms above the head while balancing along a bar

PLATE 13(b)—BELOW
Balancing along a bar

Slumped habit—tension

Expanded habit—ease

Compressed habit—tension

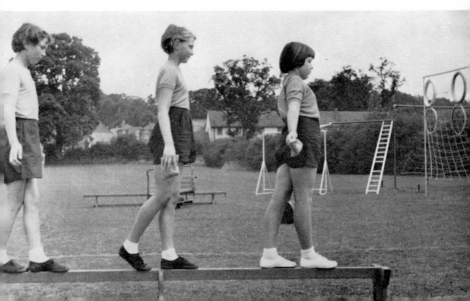

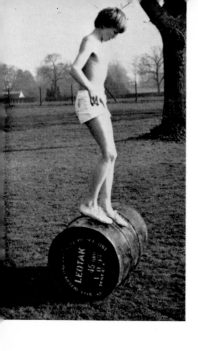
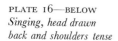

PLATE 14—LEFT
*Balancing, showing
poor use*

PLATE 15—BELOW
*Pushing, showing
sound use, wide
base of support*

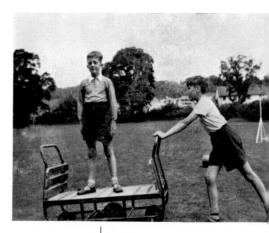

PLATE 16—BELOW
*Singing, head drawn
back and shoulders tense*

↓   ↓

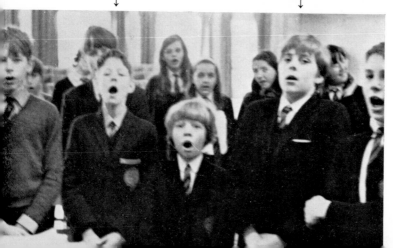

recorded amongst routine examinees . . . this proportion is undoubtedly greater than it need be as defects of this nature are very largely preventable."

The importance of early treatment of *slight* postural and other defects in children was a main theme of speakers at a special general meeting of the Research Board referred to above. Mention, too, was made of an experiment carried out at Millichope School, Shropshire. "This school was for normal, not sub-normal boys; the purpose was to find out what percentage had some defect." The experiment was really an extension of the 1948 Tottenham investigation on physical defects. Records kept of twenty-six boys, whose average age was fourteen years, showed that by the end of six months their physical deficiencies had been remedied by over 50 per cent. Though the school was small, it might well have made a unique contribution to a persistent problem. The Board hoped that their final report would be of special interest to the then Minister of Education if it proved conclusively that postural deficiencies could be cured by expert treatment.

An enquiry by two doctors on behalf of the Medical Officer to the then Board of Education, revealed the fact that 75 per cent of the children examined showed some deviation or other from good posture. This figure was also quoted in the Ministry's 1933 Syllabus of Physical Training. Admittedly the last figures refer to nearly forty years ago, but the fact is that the situation has not improved.

Dr. Wilfred Barlow, addressing the Chartered Society of Physiotherapy in 1955, said:

"Most of us I think are thoroughly dissatisfied with the results of posture training, whether it be carried out by the physical educationists or as remedial work. The incidence of defects in so-called 'normals' is tremendous. The White House Conference put it as high as 75 per cent of adolescents; my own figure, based on over 500 students and members of the Armed Services, male and female, is higher than this."

Dr. Barlow stated the crux of the problem when he continued:

"Of those who do make some initial improvement during

C

the usual posture training, very few seem to want to maintain it after supervision has been stopped. This is partly because the wrong things are taught, and partly because of a quite wrong conception of the actual training process—the accent usually being on instructing the pupil, instead of on how he is to learn something new. It is one thing to be instructed; quite another to change habit and learn."

3. ARMY RECRUITS

Although it was possible to gain some idea of the physique of school children up to the age of fifteen, it was not so easy to ascertain the position of the young worker at eighteen, and there is little available data on the physical condition of youths after this age. A report by the Medical Research Council on the physique of young adult males which was published in 1949 said:

"The details of physical defects and medical history noted in the records of the various medical boards varied considerably, some boards having no entry at all under these headings, and it was decided, therefore, that these items should be omitted from the analysis."

This was unfortunate, for such a wealth of information would have been valuable for those whose task it is to devise a national scheme of physical education for this age group.

Further enquiry by the author revealed that the National Service recruits at eighteen years were medically examined by civilian doctors on regional boards. These doctors may or may not have kept records of the physical condition of examinees. In any case, as with the Medical Research Council's report mentioned above, there was much variation in the completion of the forms, especially concerning the postural defects found. Recruits as a rule were either passed for Service or rejected. The records are scattered all over the country and are not available at any one central office. In any case, with the ending of National Service this source of examining the physical condition of young adults on a national scale, disappeared.

When a senior physical education official in the armed

services was asked by the author: "was there any evidence of common weaknesses in muscular groups or postural defects found in the military service intakes which might be a guide in determining the sort of physical training needed in further education?"; his reply was that there had been found "bad posture, in the main of a kyphosis nature (round shoulders) and to a lesser degree of a scoliosis nature (lateral curvature)." He also mentioned that shallow breathing was found, possibly due to bad posture creating too great a dependence on the diaphragm, and that there was some thoracic breathing, possibly due to weak abdominal muscles, caused through lordosis (hollow back). There was general weakness of the abdominal muscles, and general weakness of the shoulder girdle and heaving muscles.

He also said that the Medical Officer agreed with his observations and had added some further medical defects found in National Service intakes.

(a) Defects of the foot. Defects of the feet are, of course, commonly caused by faulty posture or bad footwear, and the Medical Officer had agreed that bad posture was the main cause.

(b) Poor exercise tolerance. There was a general lack of the quality of endurance.

His final comment has as much validity today as when it was written:

"It would seem from the above that the general muscular weakness of the 18-year-old could be improved if more effort were made to correct posture and the faults of breathing throughout school age and thereby improve the general physical standard of the young of today."

4. FINDINGS OF THE INDUSTRIAL WELFARE SOCIETY AND THE MINISTRY OF LABOUR

A large proportion of children do not lift in an economical and safe manner. Yet it has been proved by the work of the Industrial Welfare Society and the Central Council of Physical

Recreation that the accident rate in industry, caused by bad handling and lifting can be effectively reduced in firms where corrective training has been introduced.

"When the effects, on industrial efficiency, of nervous tension and muscular over-tension are added up, the sum, in terms of loss of production and waste, as well as human misery, must be staggering."[6] Firms wisely spend large sums on time and motion study to streamline production methods and layout. The success of such study is undeniable and has come to be accepted as part of the scientific approach to industrial problems. Even experienced workers often make many unnecessary and unrhythmical movements. Some of the movements are caused by bad placing of the apparatus used. In one factory the output of work was increased by 266 per cent when the parts to be assembled were arranged in a definite and convenient order. Analysis of the unnecessary movements does show that skilled workers make fewer movements than unskilled workers and that these movements are also more rhythmical.

In the work described in this book, the child or adult is approached in a similar way—he is examined in action, and the superfluous movements and the quite disproportionate effort to the task in hand, as well as the arrangement of the parts of his body which cause unnecessary stress, are observed and treated.

A summary of the occupational activities performed *regularly* by boys between fifteen and eighteen years of age, analysed from a sample of 1,100 boys covering all the industries and areas mentioned in a Ministry of Labour publication in the early 1960s, with percentages commensurate with figures available, was as follows:

Position or movement	Percentage of boys	
G Standing upright	66·0	⎫
Standing stooped	58·0	⎬ 81·3% on their feet
Strolling	26·2	⎭ most of day
Seated	31·3	
Kneeling	10·0	
Lying Down (mining)	3·0	
D Cycling	45·0	
Walking	65·0	

Position or movement		Percentage of boys	
E	Wearing boots	25·3	
H	1. Pushing	3·3	20% do both
	2. Pulling	4·3	
	3. Lifting (a) off bench	5·3	30% do both
	(b) off ground	12·8	
	4. Carrying (a) two hands	28·6	
	(b) one hand	10·4	
	(c) on back	6·5	33·6% carry
	(d) in front	9·5	
	(e) on shoulder	11·2	
	5. Bending (a) downwards	41·0	
	(b) sideways	0·5	52% bend
	(c) backwards	—	
	6. Digging, etc.	5·3	
	7. Reaching above the head	20·0	
	8. Sawing, etc.	31·0	
	9. Climbing (a) legs and hands	14·0	
	(b) legs only	33·0	39% climb
	(c) hands only	2·0	
	10. Hammering (a) one hand	32·0	
	(b) two hands, large hammer	1·0	38% do both
	11. Fingers (a) two hands	73·0	82% use both
	(b) one hand	8·7	
	12. Wrists (a) two hands	67·4	75% use both
	(b) one hand	7·9	

The basic material in any scheme of physical education should include sufficient activity of a suppling nature to create the mobility and flexible joint movement needed for efficient mechanical use. There is a place, too, for strengthening activities, and there should be material to counteract any postural weaknesses—all to help develop and maintain the most efficient individual posture. This material can be incorporated quite naturally into the increasing number of activities found in the options for senior students at school or college during recent years, for example, archery, canoeing, horse riding, rock climbing and skating.

To give a detailed account of the effects of these activities would necessitate examination of the young people on the spot and over a period of time. This was unnecessary for the purpose here, but interpretation of the percentages does give a general picture of the movements youths perform at work and their possible effects.

5. CONCLUSIONS

Looking at the Summary's findings, several points may be made.

(a) *Possible suppling or mobility tendencies.* Few of the movements appear likely to give much mobility, and none is performed by the whole age group. Cycling (45 per cent) may aid mobility of the knee and hip. Over 40 per cent of the boys performed a bending downward movement regularly, which may help mobility of the hip joint, although it gives little or no abduction of the joint. Only 20 per cent ever reach above the head. Special emphasis should therefore be paid to activities demanding full-range mobility of the joints and spine, to encourage the development of sound mechanical use.

(b) *Possible strengthening tendencies.*

There are no potentially strengthening activities performed regularly by the whole group. Those that might be included in this category for toning-up the larger muscle groups (cycling 45 per cent, lifting 30 per cent, carrying 33 per cent, digging 5 per cent, climbing 39 per cent) are performed by a third or less of the youths. A sound scheme therefore requires all-round muscle toning games and activities using all the main muscle groups.

(c) *Possible postural tendencies.*

Approximately half of the activities (*see* lines 1–12 in Fig. 4) may be likely to produce some degree of kyphosis, unless performed with sound use.

CHAPTER 3

Daily Occupations and Adult Posture

The Stance of the Worker

There is a connection between osteo–arthritis and bodily misuse. A pastry cook's habitual posture for over twenty years was standing stooped with a slight twist to the left in the lumbar spine.[7] With a repeated single movement, he stamped out pastry from a strip which was carried past him on a conveyor belt. The X-ray of his lumbar spine showed the development of an osteophytic outgrowth at the precise spot where he made the twist.

Another example demonstrated how a dentist's stance for his entire working life had thrown severe strain on the cervical (neck) spine, creating osteo–arthritis in this region.[8] His position bending over a patient showed gross dorsal kyphosis and accentuated cervical curve, with head retraction and braced knees which led to osteo–arthritic changes and disc degeneration on very much the same lines as the pastry cook. If only he had bent at the hips and flexed his knees or used a swivel stool to lower the body and still keep the trunk aligned much pain and inconvenience might have been prevented.

Quite recently electromyographic techniques have made it clear that muscular over–activity occurs in many patients complaining of anxiety and tension. There is also an intimate relationship between states of anxiety and observable states of muscular tension.

One author in an exhaustive book on "Headaches" found[9] that by far the largest group of any patients was made up of those with "marked contraction in the muscles of the neck . . . and common are the sustained contractions associated with emotional strain, dissatisfaction, apprehension and anxiety."

A photograph of a typical patient who suffered from chronic head pains associated with anxiety, showed tense trapezii muscles in the neck, raised shoulders and buttock tension.[10] A

later photograph, taken after he had learnt to relax this unnecessary tension and was free from head pains and anxiety
showed that tension had been released in the neck, shoulder
and buttocks, and that he has gained in height and shoulder
breadth (*see* Fig. 7).

A civil servant had severe cervical spondylosis (a fusing of
the neck vertebrae) with an associated brachial neuralgia.[11] It
was possible to train him to release the tension which was
deforming his posture, and in this position he was free from
pain. Such, however, was his engrained attitude of cringing in
front of his superior that he was unable to maintain the improved posture until he eventually had had a row with his boss.

Such deforming attitudes of cringing and evasiveness eventually lead to structural change; the evasive action of turning
the gaze away by rotating the head will often set up a marked
scoliosis in the cervico-dorsal (neck) junction.

The Stance of the Athlete

The javelin and ball thrower have already been mentioned
in Chapter 1. Another case is that of a young acrobatic dancer
who had a slight lateral curvature of the spine which caused
her pain and prevented her from working.[12] (It should be
noted that postural deformities may be painless, provided that
stress activities are avoided, but this involves an increasing
limitation of the individual's range of activities.) In spite of
long treatment by static holding and contraction exercises, the
dancer was still in pain and it could be seen on film that when
she did her backbend, her deformity *increased* considerably. She
was quite unaware of this deformity.

An assiduous "body builder" with a lateral curvature in his
neck and with an habitually raised left shoulder, increased his
pain and deformity by his exercises.[13] The trend to introduce
"weight training" into all forms of sport and into schools has
its dangers in this respect. The added weight creates a stress
situation, which, as with the acrobatic dancer and the body
builder, increases any fault there is and quickly brings out
any latent postural weakness.

Unless children and young people start with sound postural

habits, exercises can do more harm than good. This is especially the case with passive and static spanning exercises of various kinds and with exercises that press the head backward. In addition to compressing and crushing the spine, as with the typical arch-spanning movement of the hysteric, they interfere with the proper functioning of the body and affect posture. These contraction exercises have been thought to "strengthen the back muscles" but this is based on a faulty conception of "strength."[14] Inman (1952) has shown that the longer the resting length of a muscle, the greater the force exerted and the less the electro-myographic activity which accompanies it. The "strength" to maintain adequate postural relationships at rest and during movement does not come from muscle-shortening and over-contraction, but from maintaining a correct equilibrium between the various parts of the body. To attain this equilibrium, the patient needs to be taught to release superfluous muscular tension and return to a resting state in which the muscles are lengthening."[15]

CHAPTER 4

How to achieve Good Posture

How then, can we help to look after ourselves, and make good use of our bodies?

Definitions of Posture

The popular conception of posture as "how a person stands and walks" is vague and inadequate, and it gives no hint of how vital a person's posture is to his effectiveness, well-being and enjoyment.

It is therefore necessary to define posture. A comprehensive definition (and one which shows that mind, body and habit have their parts to play) is "a person's willingness and ability to maintain that relationship of the different parts of his body which ensures their most efficient behavioural function and physiological functioning both now and in the future."[16]

The effectiveness of an action, the absence of inappropriate muscular tensions, and the grace and poise with which it is executed are inseparable and are dependent upon the body being well arranged at the beginning and throughout the action. Broadly speaking, there are three states of posture, although the same person can display them all at any one time: slumped, contracted and expanded (*see* Fig. 5 and Plate 13).

The "slumped," floppy or slack state where some of the muscles are not active enough to secure a good mechanical arrangement of the body leads to strain in other muscles and to a strain on the joints when in action. For example, if a "floppy" person lifts a heavy weight he is more likely to strain his back and other joints than the person with good postural tone.

In the "contracted" postural state parts of the body, such as the ribs, may be fixed and immobilised and there is an undue pulling in of joint surfaces upon each other, for example in the neck and shoulders.

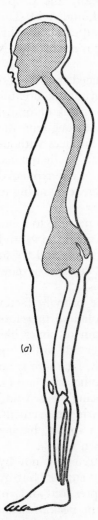
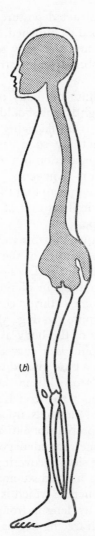
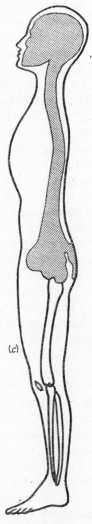

(*a*) Slumped habit, sagging with braced knees.

(*b*) Expanded habit, when the body is lightly eased-up.

(*c*) Contracted habit, causing compression right along the column, limiting chest movement and adding to joint strain.

FIG. 5—*Let the spine lengthen all the time.*

The variations of contracted posture are many and people displaying it are described as hunched, braced, and rigid. The muscles are over-active and the body tense and crushed. This also leads to strain, disturbs and restricts movement and is wasteful of energy.

In the "expanded" state the body is balanced, poised and alert, the head carried lightly, the shoulder buoyant, the breathing unrestricted. There is no flaccidity in the trunk or limbs, but rather muscular activity so distributed throughout the body as to allow light separation of the joint surfaces without putting undue strain on connecting muscles or ligaments. "Expanded" tone does not mean that the muscles are expanded like a balloon, a better simile is that of a sponge, expanding to its natural size and shape.

Using the word "posture" in this way, it is possible to think meaningfully about the posture of the spine, arm, hand and even finger. (Pull in the joint surfaces of the fingers and try to write.) This habitual pulling in of the joint surfaces is now recognised as cause of some arthritic conditions.

The posture of the spine (*see* Fig. 5) is the primary factor determining the posture of the body as a whole and therefore its performance. The spine is a curved column of bones like cotton-reels arising from a base jointed on either side to the hip bones. In one sense it "grows" from the pelvis, for there is no mechanism within the body to "stretch" the spine (*see* Plate 1). Co-ordinated movement depends upon it being "eased-up" throughout its length, preparatory to and during movement. This "easing-up" is somewhat analagous to a spring, having been freed from compression, recovering its own length.

This postural state is arrived at not by stretching nor by attempts to flatten a structure which is rightly curved, but by freeing it throughout its length from compression and an imbalance of pulls. Such freeing begins with the neck muscles, so that the head is in no way pulled in upon the spine (*see* Fig. 6).

An improvement in the habitual neck, head and
spine relationship is basic to the better use and
management of the body.

When the living spine is free from compression, postural

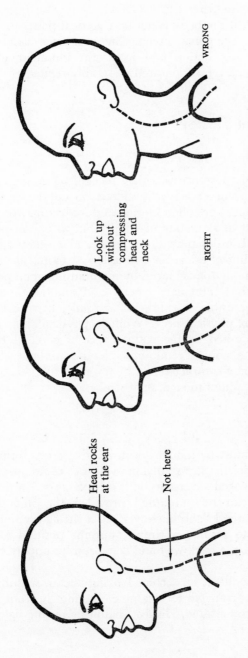

Look up without compressing head and neck

RIGHT

WRONG

Head rocks at the ear

Not here

FIG. 6—*The relationship of the* HEAD, NECK *and* SPINE *is fundamental to sound posture, it is the* PRIMARY CONTROL. *Observe people, and visualise the neck spine, starting at the ear and passing through the centre of the shoulder. Is it expanded or contracted?*

reflexes operate to bring it to a state which may be described as "eased-up" or, if the body is not in a vertical position, "eased outward" from the pelvis. Freeing the spine from compression implies dispersing undue and irrelevant muscular tension, since posture and relaxation are inseparably related.

Relaxation and Tension

1. ITS NATURE

Though its importance is widely recognised nowadays, the nature of relaxation is not always understood and the techniques for its achievement are often limited and misleading. It should not be thought of as a state of "flop," but as one of proportionate effort. It is dynamic, not negative. There should be just the right amount of effort for the task—no more, no less. In action this can only be achieved by maintaining good posture.

Relaxation has muscular, mental and emotional aspects, which are inseparable. A child, for example, can be unduly tense because of physical stress. While in physical effort undue tension is minimised by the maintenance of good posture in action, in mental effort it is minimised by the child not allowing himself to become contracted and by not restricting his breathing. This also applies to emotional stresses.

2. RELAXATION EXERCISES

Relaxation must be thought of in relative terms, of course, for given sufficient stress anyone will be come disturbed. Mentally provoked over-tension, or example, during an examination, can be minimised provided the student has previously practised "checking-over" in a sitting position. It is best for him to assume a simple, upright position for this procedure with the back well and comfortably supported.

(a) He should sit on a chair looking ahead, with his legs comfortably arranged, for example, one foot in front of the other or ankles crossed. His feet should be resting lightly on the floor.

(*b*) He should be aware of what is in front of him without fixing the eyes or staring.

(*c*) He should attend to his neck, head and trunk, in that order, with the idea of letting the neck ease so that the head is lightly poised and the spinal column can ease up throughout its curves. (This "easing-up" is the principal factor determining the body's posture and is the desirable constant in the management of body.)

(*d*) The student should now attend to his shoulders, abdomen and rib-cage with the idea of letting the shoulders rest lightly and of letting the stomach and chest move freely, without restriction or exaggeration.

(*e*) He should refresh some awareness of the body as a whole, supported on the chair, and using "the thought of a smile" as a guide to the direction in which the muscles of the head and face can ease. This easing can pervade the whole body, and with practice a child, a student or a teacher can achieve a more expanded state of posture at will, with the result that it gradually becomes the habitual state.

A similar relaxation procedure can also be used for the emotionally provoked tension of self-consciousness, but it must be emphasised that the skill necessary to minimise these two kinds of tension must be learned beforehand. A child or a student cannot wait until the stress situation has arisen to apply the remedy.

It is suggested to students in training that if during their ordinary lectures (and without withdrawing their attention from the lecturer) they developed this habit of checking-over their bodies, they would better be able to remain cool, calm and collected during an examination, in front of a class, or at a party.

3. "EASING-UP"

The following procedure is suggested to teachers as a means of easing-up after a tiring day or as a preparation for sleep for those students and teachers who find it difficult to "let-up."

To relax lying down the student should lie on the floor, which being hard will enable him to detect tension which is disguised on a soft bed. He should lie on a rug or a folded blanket, avoiding a draught. If he is round-shouldered he should rest his head on a book just thick enough to prevent the head falling back.

He should then either flex his knees comfortably or put something firm under his thighs—a rolled-up mat will do—especially if he has big hips or a hollow back. His arms should rest by his sides or, if he prefers it, his fingers should be folded lightly over his abdomen. His eyes should be closed.

(*a*) He should remind himself that for a while other things can wait, that for a short time there is nothing to do.

(*b*) He should sense that the whole of his body—his head, trunk, arms and legs—is supported by the floor, that he can give himself completely to the floor for support. He should realise that he is borne as securely by the floor as a log is borne on water when it floats.

(*c*) He should feel the floor against all the areas of his body that it touches: the back of the head, the upper part of the back, the arms, legs and heels. He can feel this contact without pressing down and as he does so he should have the idea of letting them ease, soften and spread.

(*d*) He should let his attention move, with a gentle and steady shifting of focus throughout his shoulders and arms and legs. He must not hold on to them and he should accompany this shifting of attention (which is like the moving beam of a torch) with the idea of allowing any tension to disperse and the muscles to soften and ease, *even if they feel released*. This is especially important, for what *feels* released may not be released at all. He should do the same with his neck so that he is not holding on to his head and his throat is open and free. (It is often over-contracted in singing or talking—*see* Plate 16.)

(*e*) He should let his tongue rest and allow his face and jaw muscles to ease in the direction of a smile. This is an easy "unmasked," unstrained and pleasant attitude, which he should allow to spread throughout his whole body.

(*f*) Directing his attention to the movement of his ribs and abdomen, he should allow these to take place without restriction or exaggeration.

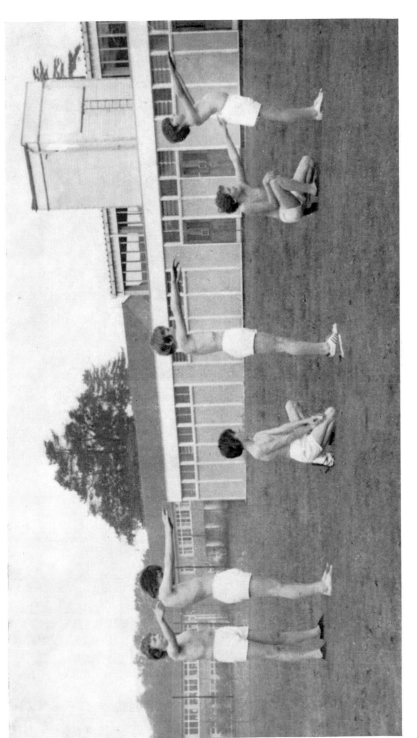

PLATE 17
Checking in pairs

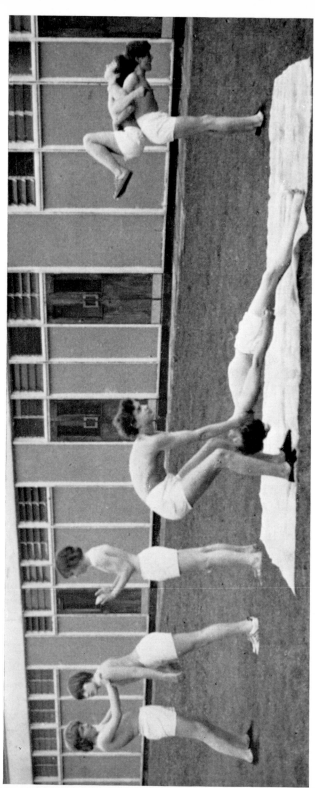

Rocking the dummy with poor use

Lifting the log with poor mechanical performance and use

Lifting the sack with poor performance and strain

PLATE 18(a)

Three recreational activities: little attention has been paid to performance

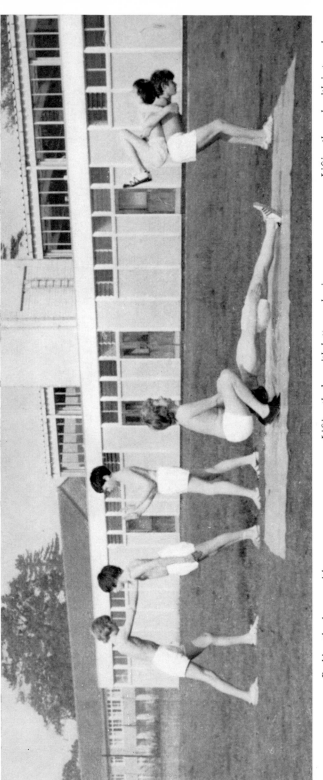

Rocking the dummy with
better support

Lifting the log with better mechanics
but not really good use, e.g. lifter
has heels off ground, head drawn back

Lifting the sack with improved
use, knees flexed

PLATE 18 (b)

Three recreational activities: stress has been placed by the teacher on mechanics and
use, and all activities show improved mechanical performance

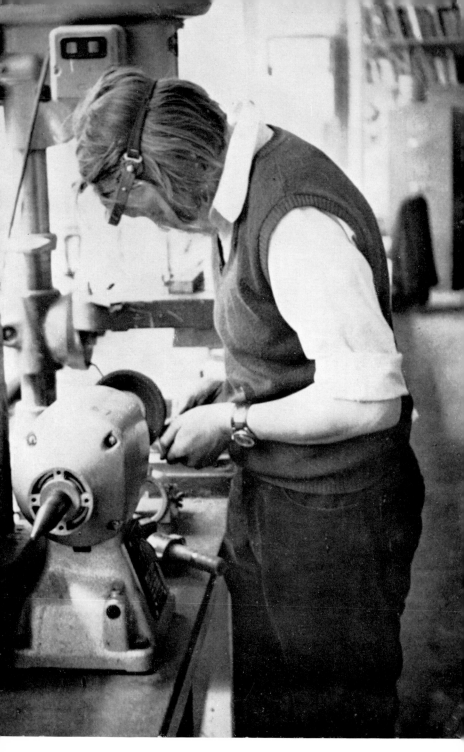

PLATE 19
Working at the lathe: position of strain (see Plate 20)

(g) By now he should be able to refresh the sense of his body as a whole, supported throughout, in an easy open attitude, effortlessly breathing.

(h) Finally, he should stretch! An easy, enjoyable, cat-like stretch right throughout the body—and then he should slowly get up. (This stretch is important to bring back sufficient muscle tone for standing.)

4. DISPERSING TENSION

The accomplishment of real relaxation come from *doing it,* even if at first, for some people, little result is apparent. Everyone gets tense under certain circumstances and, by the end of a working day, most people have accumulated and carry with them muscular activity that has nothing to do with meeting the needs of sitting on the bus going home or feeding at the meal table. Once a teacher, a student or a child has learned to disperse unneeded tenseness at will, he has gained a most valuable and worthwhile accomplishment.

We should try to remember the procedure for getting rid of unnecessary tenseness—it has a beginning, a middle, and an end. We should practise methodically for a few minutes at a time, though we will find that our attention wanders and that from time to time we get lost in thought or day-dreams. This is everyone's experience and when a teacher or a student notices it, he must simply bring his attention back and carry on.

All these instructions simply mean "relax;" but by doing it in this particular way the total amount and quality of the attention one can sustain are greater and consequently more effective. When first learning to relax it is both useful and important deliberately to tense the arms and legs and then let go the tension just created.

To do this, the teacher or the student simply attends to his arms and legs, experiencing the tenseness created, with the idea in mind of letting it disperse. He does not need to move, nor to fix the arms and legs in positions, nor to think "concentratedly" on them, nor to "think them heavy." He simply attends to them, sensing them in so far as he can with the idea in mind of permitting them to be at ease. This brings out the fundamental and familiar point in relaxation: the amount of

D

tenseness that is habitual feels right, feels even released, yet very often is not so, for there is a certain amount of unnecessary muscular activity of which the student or the teacher is not aware because it is habitual. That is why, after releasing the tenseness he has deliberately created, he should continue to attend to his arms and legs with the idea of further possible release in the direction just experienced. In this way it is sometimes possible to "get though" to tension below the threshold of awareness.

As the teacher or student does this, the resulting sensory experience may be slightly unfamiliar. He should be quite prepared for this, take an interest in the fact and accept it, for through his training he has the means of gaining a new appreciation of his body as an instrument capable of skilled use.

Once the student gets the general idea of what tension is, it is not necessary deliberately to stiffen for a start, so long as he remembers that with tension, as with an iceberg, a certain proportion is out of sight, below the threshold of awareness.

He may prefer to think of release (the thing he wishes to allow) as a softening, a spreading, or an expanding. Sometimes to have an analogy at the back of the mind can help greatly. One of the best of these is that of the sponge, for when it is freed from squeezing it gradually comes to its own shape and bulk, light and open in texture.

Analogies may or may not help, but it is important that the student is clear on what he is setting about. He is attending methodically to his body, letting his attention move throughout it with the idea of permitting release. If on any occasion there is release, well and good; if there is not, he should be content for he has done all that there is to be done in this way to effect it. Accomplishment, as in many other fields of activity, can only come with time and practice.

Directing Attention

This activity called "directing attention" is so basic to relaxation that it is worth saying a little more about it. Experience has shown that the best attitude to adopt when relaxing by directing attention is "a questing" one. The student assumes that he cannot sense one iota of what there is to sense. He embarks upon an exploration—in the dark, and with a weak battered torch. He moves his attention through part after part of the body, "getting in close," and assuming all the time that there may be much more than he can discern. He does all this searching almost casually, yet steadily and with interest, but without building up that fixity popularly associated with concentrating or "getting down to it." It is attention without tension; a gently shifting focus without straining for results and certainties.

Results come when least sought after; they come through an ever-improving quality of attention. Just after practising the lying-down sequence, the student should notice that in those movements it is possible to be very wide awake, bright, alert and completely at peace with himself. It is a fallacy that to get better concentration he must fix his head, frown his brows and screw up his eyes. The reverse is the truth, for these muscular fixities impair and diminish his powers of attention. When he is relaxed in the way described above, that is, in the expanded state of the posture which involves balance, light tone and poise, he is at his most receptive, and he will learn, enjoy and appreciate most readily. Recognition of this increased receptivity as an aid to learning is important to all education and not only to physical education.

Thus from the educational as well as from the physical point of view, school should be the obvious place to train children as early as possible in the techniques of this approach to relaxation. From the moment they start school at five "directing attention" to the use of their bodies should be developed as a normal and habitual approach to learning.

Irrelevant Tension

In relaxation, undue tension can usefully be described as activity irrelevant to the job in hand. Relaxation involves *appropriate* effort. The pupil is relaxed in work or play when he is exerting the effort needed for what he is doing; no more and no less.

Muscular tension when lying down needs to be very little

because there is negligible activity apart from breathing, which itself is slight. Relaxing is usually thought of as "taking it easy" in this way. But children have to be taught to relax when lying down. This may seem surprising since it might be supposed that in such a position there was no other possibility than to be relaxed. This is not so, for the amount of tension the child habitually has in his body in this position feels right, feels even relaxed, but in fact is not. There is usually an amount of irrelevant tension of which the child is not aware. With guidance, however, he can "get through" to a deeper relaxation than he customarily experiences.

It is of very great importance to ensure that children are taught to stretch and move before rising from relaxation. They may have started with too much tension "in the wrong direction," but the state of muscular tone they reach (which is appropriate to lying down) is by no means appropriate for movement, even the movement of rising again. Therefore they stretch and move their limbs so that the muscular tone increases, but this time it is more balanced and distributed throughout their bodies.

If there is too little tone (flaccidity), it is not enough to maintain the body's good arrangement. Posture is disturbed, the condition for co-ordinated movement is disturbed. To be relaxed in sitting or standing, for example, the muscles should be able to maintain the "expanded" state of posture described above.

Conversely, if the posture is disturbed by bracing the shoulders or legs by "tummy-tightness" that locks the ribs and breathing, it is clearly not a relaxed state. Once again posture, movement and relaxation are inseparately related.

It follows, therefore, that boys and girls cannot be shown how to use their bodies better if they approach the task unduly tense. Relaxation is no mere prescription for a sick or nervous child—it is the condition in which boys and girls are at their most alert and receptive. It is the state in which they can learn most readily and easily, and in which they can give of their best. In physical education it is a pre-requisite of improving habits of movement. If the child is unduly tense, which is the normal state in human beings, he cannot choose the way he will do a job. For example, if he sings by drawing the head backward and downward and poking out the chin, he is caught up in this habit unless he can reform it starting from rest (*see* Plate 16).

It is not enough just to point out a faulty habit. When the pupil is encouraged first to come to rest, free from any effort not required for sitting, he is ready to begin to appreciate the preparatory tensing of the body and limbs *at the thought of singing or writing*. By being encouraged to come to rest again and again, and to choose a different means of setting about the task, he will be able to alter the injurious habit.

Posture, then, is primary. A clear intention is formed and carried through with gradually increasing accomplishment so long as in the learning stages the aim is to maintain posture throughout, making the task secondary.

Practising Relaxation

There are several exercises that can be performed which are useful in themselves, but only so far as they enable us to be much more observant of ourselves in everyday activities so that we can sense when we are tense and do something about it.

To develop a kinaesthetic sense of the difference between muscular contractions and relaxations by using separate muscle groups and observing the actions taking place the child or adult should:

(*a*) Grip his pen or pencil strongly while writing, then release as much muscular tension as he can and still be able to write. He should try the same thing with other small articles like a piece of chalk, a crayon, a rubber and a pair of knitting needles.

(*b*) Grip his right forearm with his left hand, alternately clench his fist and "let go" to feel his forearm muscles contract and relax. Next he should hold out his fingers alternately stretching them straight and tense and letting go as the hand softly closes. He should clench his fist and notice what happens to his elbow and shoulder. Trying an arm swinging movement with his fist clenched, notice how the flow of movement is impeded.

(c) Place his left hand over the front of his right upper arm, alternately turn the palm of his right hand to face up and then down.

(d) Place his left hand over the tip of his right shoulder, raise the entire arm upward and away from the side and then let it "fall" relaxed. Repeating this, he should lower it slowly to demonstrate controlled movement. Relaxing his arm to the side again, he should try and eliminate all controlled movement. He should continue to practise until his arm dangles without any apparent voluntary control.

(e) Hold his hands in position over the piano or the desk, alternatively raise his elbows away from his sides and then let them fall relaxed.

(f) Shrugging or raising the shoulders and relaxing he should notice whether both shoulders are level. Quite frequently one shoulder is held higher than the other—more often than not through habit. It is in fact quite a common fault that shoulders are normally "held" in a position much

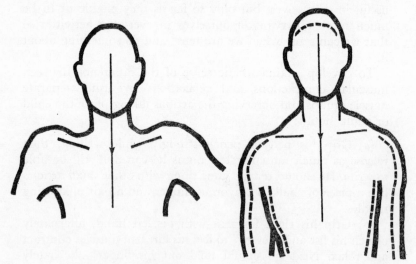

(a) Shoulders habitually HELD up, causing continual tension, often resulting in shoulder and neck pain and restricted breathing.

(b) By releasing the spine throughout its length and releasing unnecessary tension, height and shoulder breadth increase.

FIG. 7—The position of the shoulders.

higher than they should be (*see* Fig. 7). The child should be taught to let them hang lightly. But he may be so tense that considerable time is required before residual tensions are relaxed and the shoulders are lowered and equalised.

(*g*) The child should straighten upward in the sitting position as tall and as tense as possible before relaxing his neck muscles and allowing his head to slump forward. He should then continue to relax his back muscles, allowing his body to slump forward and gradually straighten, tensing again, and then repeat by relaxing.

(*h*) Resting both feet on the floor with no great pressure on the thighs he should place his hands in his lap, raise his feet forwards off the floor and feel his thigh muscles tensing. Lowering, keeping tense and then relaxing he should feel his muscles letting go.

(*i*) Observe facial tensions by frowning, wrinkling the forehead, closing the eyes tightly, puckering the lips and screwing up the nose. Then, in the manner described above, no longer emphasise these tensions, but relax them by imagining the head to be a sponge, which has been squeezed tightly. "Let go" and "think a smile."

(*j*) Assuming the correct position of the hands for writing, drawing, playing the piano or the recorder, tense the fingers by straightening them stiffly and then relax them by letting go (*see* Plate 11). Extend the hands at the wrists or raise the hands upwards and then relax them by letting them drop. It is well to remember that the rest of his body should be checked when performing such activities, for pianists and typists, for example, very often get neck and back pains through unnecessary muscle contraction.

It should be remembered that when a person is writing, reading, eating, driving, typing or performing many other tasks in a sitting position the leg muscles are quite often kept unnecessarily tense. Driving a car reveals the anxieties and emotions which create tension; for example, the calf and thigh muscles of the accelerator leg often become over-tensed when passing another car, and the neck muscles are tightened and the back hollowed if a cat suddenly darts across the road, and this is only natural. But the driver should be aware of it and he should not hang on to the tension after the incident; he should ease off, let go, and get back to the normal relaxed sitting position.

The child should be allowed to experiment with his movements through the full range of activities. When, for example, he knows from his simple lessons in anatomy that the head pivots from a point approximately between the ears, he should be allowed to feel and try out movement from that point, for many children (and adults) believe falsely that the head moves from the knob at the back of the neck.

CHAPTER 5

Teaching Good Habit in Schools—I

Changes in Approach to Physical Education

Though the history of games and sports in Great Britain goes back many hundreds of years, the introduction of gymnastics teaching on a national scale is a comparatively recent innovation, beginning only early in the present century.

In 1871, the Board of Education had advised school managers who wished to have their boys "drilled" to make the best arrangements they could, and they had also suggested rates of pay for army instructors who visited schools for this purpose; although twenty years later the Board had substituted "physical exercises" for the word "drill", their regulations were still based very largely on military handbooks.

Despite many attempts to introduce less military and more educationally sound methods of physical education into schools, it was not until a new syllabus was published after the First World War that the formal nature of the lessons was reduced to a minimum and every effort made to make P.T. more interesting and enjoyable.

Following the publication of another and more famous syllabus in 1933, the old, narrow and rigid "school drill" disappeared, and its place was taken by exercises adapted to meet the varying needs and capabilities of children of different ages. Freer movements and more purposeful activities replaced the old military exercises, and greater use was made of movements based on the natural rhythms of the body, which assisted joint mobility and general muscular tone. They also helped to encourage a more relaxed, less tense attitude generally.

Later developments in physical training were mainly improvements in methods, exercises and apparatus, the exercises designed to encourage all-round bodily and remedial activity, and the apparatus to develop independence, courage, agility and physical skill.

47

Methods of teaching became more natural and interesting, greater use being made of many and smaller groups of children. The words of command were framed to ensure mental activity before physical response, and the instructor's bark was silenced.

Twenty years after its publication, the 1933 syllabus was replaced by two books: *Moving and Growing*—a short study of the movement of growing children, and *Planning the Programme*—which is concerned with physical education in the primary school.

Like every other subject, physical education has changed considerably even since 1953. For the teacher today it should be the study of the management of the body, a study of all that is meant by the words posture, movement and tension (including nervous tension) at work and in play, in sport and at school.

The physical training lesson must be treated, therefore, in the same way as any other practical lesson. To get the best results the classes should be as small as they are for woodwork, housecraft and other practical subjects, and by means of group work and individual attention children should have the opportunity of developing their physical skills according to their own needs and at their own rate.

Education and Posture

The idea that special attention should be given to those children who are physically backward is already influencing physical education, and many children are being given the chance of building up strength and skill in movement.

"One cannot help but feel," commented an official writer on the health of the school child in 1956, "that there is a tendency in school to encourage the child who has a natural aptitude for physical games and activities at the expense of his fellow who does not share his enthusiasm. While one could not hope nor expect to see children graded intellectually, I should like to see the physically backward receive that little extra attention and encouragement they so badly need."

True as it may be that there is a significant proportion of

children with observable defects, there are an even greater number who do not manage themselves in the most economical way. It is, therefore, both advisable and reasonable that all children should be given the opportunity of developing postural skills and sound body mechanics in order to prevent the complaints which can develop later in life through faulty use of the body.

"In the past a great deal of attention has been given in school to methods of imparting knowledge; very little has been given to methods of developing skilled movements, yet the importance of muscular skill in promoting mental as well as physical health has been impressively demonstrated by F. M. Alexander."[2] In physical education, the pendulum has swung away from the rigidity of the old-style drill to an emphasis on physical re-creation.

In future, the emphasis will be towards making children more aware of the way they perform their movements in the classroom and on the playing field, and making them realise that they can use their bodies skilfully or clumsily, a task which involves paying as much attention to *how* activities are done as to *what* is being done.

It will come to be recognised that the management of a person's body depends on how he stands, sits, walks, sleeps, speaks and works, rather than on whether he has some daily exercise or plays a game, for experience has shown that even the ordinary everyday things which a person does can affect the well-being of his body.

Whatever daily, occupational or athletic activities children and adults have to perform, all the evidence shows that unless they are based upon sound postural habits they lead to pain, inefficiency, damage and defects, which may become serious.

When the body is used correctly, there is no strain on any part, physical and mental processes are at their best and the personality of the individual is able to shine through.

The fundamental aim in education and training for better body mechanics and posture should be the attainment of a greater degree of efficiency. This efficiency depends upon the principles of balance, the flexibility of the joints, and good mechanical use of all parts of the body, especially of the upper and lower extremities.

It is also well to remember that each child's body is peculiar to him and he must find the arrangement of the skeletal framework best suited to himself. What is applicable for one child is not necessarily so for another, although, of course, there are certain fundamental principles common to all. It is not possible, therefore, to give a few exercises which can be carried out by everybody. To do so might well cause harm to some.

Let it be quite clearly understood that there is no suggestion here of omitting any aspect of physical education or any of the beneficial games, sports or gymnastics already in use in our schools. Rather it is an attempt *to improve the management of the body when engaged in these activities*. The physical educationalist realises that although it may strengthen specific muscle groups, piecemeal exercising does not lead to more graceful or more effective movement and co-ordination.

Contrary to some opinions, it is possible to improve movement quality in general by developing a sound posture which can be used in any activity. The teaching of specific actions should therefore not be necessary. A child who uses himself well will demonstrate it in *any* action he cares to perform. A child with good posture will lift well naturally, but since good use of the body in many children is not spontaneous, it has to be taught, and until such teaching has become an integral part of education from the child's admission to school, there is a case for teaching specific movements (*see* Plate 4).

Practice is necessary for all actions, but practice alone will not improve a tennis or a cricket stroke if the player is, for example, too tense in the shoulder. Instead of doing separate exercises for individual muscle groups, attention should be directed to the body as a whole, by observing posture. The primary structural control of posture lies in the position of the head and spinal column relative to the rest of the body. In other words, if the head and spine are kept in the right alignment, then all the other parts tend to come into line, too, although, of course, attention must be paid to specific parts as well. Certainly if the head and spinal column are badly aligned in action, the whole body will be thrown out of balance and excessive strain will be felt in some areas of the body, while other muscle groups may be given little to do. It is no satisfactory cure merely to exercise these undeveloped muscles, for this will not bring about better co-ordinated movement. The cure lies in dealing with the underlying disturbance of posture. The under-developed muscles will then tend to do their proper job and develop normally.

The new approach can be summarised by saying that pupils are considered individually and their everyday and occupational movements are observed. They are shown where their faults lie—partly visually and partly by being shown how to achieve well co-ordinated movement. The crux of postural education is this: what is habitual feels right, yet what feels right is not necessarily so at all and, in the long run, may even be injurious, as some instances have shown. Even the simple action of taking up a pencil can be a bad postural habit, wasteful of energy and impairing a child's performance and powers of attention.

The most important field for the establishment of these new methods is in the schools, where children can early be prevented from acquiring tenseness and bad habits of posture and movement. Visitors to a school in Surrey have been interested in the amount of attention being paid by the children to the way in which they do quite usual and ordinary things such as lifting, pushing and walking. They were surprised to notice a little girl seemingly quite engrossed in the mundane action of walking forward, picking something from the ground, and going across to a chair to sit on it, *an activity which includes many fundamental movements.*

This attention to the way in which ordinary things are done is a deliberate feature of the children's physical education, for they are being encouraged to use their bodies well both in class and on the field. On a modest scale, they are being given instruction in posture, movement, and the ability to be relaxed in activity.

The importance of posture to parent and teacher alike is this: when a child learns to use his body in a more co-ordinated way, it tends to function better. Training helps the child's well-being, for as he learns to approach his tasks with poise and calm his powers of attention and his performance tend to improve.

None of the beneficial trends in modern physical education are being omitted in this school, but an additional effort is being made to improve the use of the body during the games, athletics, gymnastics, swimming and dancing lessons. The teachers are trying to make the body's performance in these activities more efficient by paying attention first to *how* things are done and only second to *what* is being done.

When a violinist plays a concerto he makes use of two instruments: one is the violin and the other is his own body. It is this conception of the body as an instrument capable of increasingly skilled use, co-ordination and performance which children should appreciate. Nationally-known musicians appreciate the value of this technique applied to their work.

Children and adults should realise that they can *either* use their bodies in every kind of activity in an effective, stress-free and co-ordinated manner *or* in a way which gives poor results, is awkward and leads to strain. If boys and girls are to be taught to make the most of their potential it is necessary for their teachers to recognise the full importance of posture. This applies not only to physical education, but to all aspects of education. For it has been proved that when children become more aware of themselves in this sense their receptivity is increased, they become more alert and retentive. The time will come when all teachers, like athletes, will make use of relaxation to solve their problems. For the more relaxed a child is in activity, the longer he can carry on, the more effort he can direct to good use.

Posture and the Curriculum

Experience in a junior mixed and infant school in Surrey has shown that instruction in posture can best be fitted into the curriculum in four ways, which complement one another. First, all the children in a class can be taught a very elementary knowledge of the structure of the body and its movement. Secondly, the teacher can take one small group in turn during the group activities of the physical education lesson, whilst supervising the class as a whole. Thirdly, a few children can be given special individual attention appropriate to their difficulties and fourthly, there should be a continual check on the use being made of the body in all school activities such as gardening, games, craft, dancing, speech and writing. This check should be made in just the same way as cleanliness, tidiness or punctuality are checked in the habit-forming primary school years.

The suggestions which follow will help a child to learn good postural habits. But it must be remembered that the real meaning of these suggested activities and exercises lies in the experience gained by the pupil. Just as a games master goes on a practical course to improve his performance and does not rely on a book to increase his skill, so by experience a child will gain increasing skill in using his body. In very few people is sensory appreciation sound enough for them accurately to interpret a written or verbal instruction, and the descriptions on the following pages cannot replace practical experience with a specialist teacher.

At the present time it is presupposed that specialists in physical education are needed primarily in the secondary schools. Yet teachers well trained in postural education and the management of the body are needed above all in the infants' school, where they can lay the foundations of good use.

The infant stage is most important, because it is here that children acquire skills of all kinds, and these should be sound skills and good habits based on how things are done rather than on what is being done. As this is the time in their lives when children are experimenting with their hands a good deal, a continual check should be made to see that right from the start there is good use in the way they hold their various implements.

In the junior school (*see* Fig. 8), there will be a natural development of the "domestic" skills such as picking up, pushing, pulling, lifting, carrying and writing and of the fundamental skills of games and sports: catching, throwing, batting, dribbling, bowling, and so on. Whether performed individually or in small groups it is vital that these actions should be based on sound postural principles.

During the secondary and further education stages, the pupils can continue to practise the domestic skills in the natural conditions of games and work. Similarly, they can develop "good use" in sawing, filing, planing, typing, sewing, digging, etc., and they should learn and experience as many types of games and sports as possible. Throughout these activities

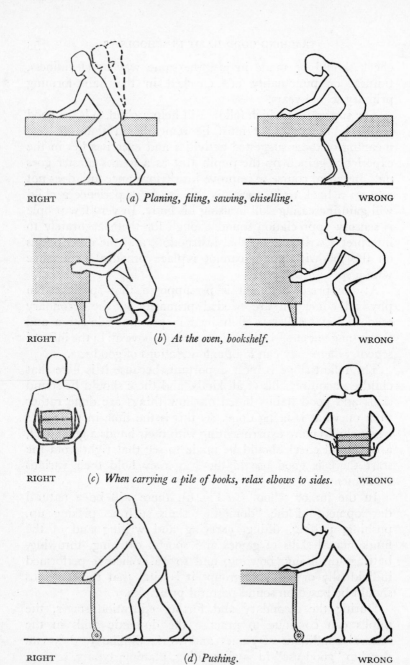

RIGHT   (a) *Planing, filing, sawing, chiselling.*   WRONG

RIGHT   (b) *At the oven, bookshelf.*   WRONG

RIGHT   (c) *When carrying a pile of books, relax elbows to sides.*   WRONG

RIGHT   (d) *Pushing.*   WRONG

FIG. 8—*School activities.*

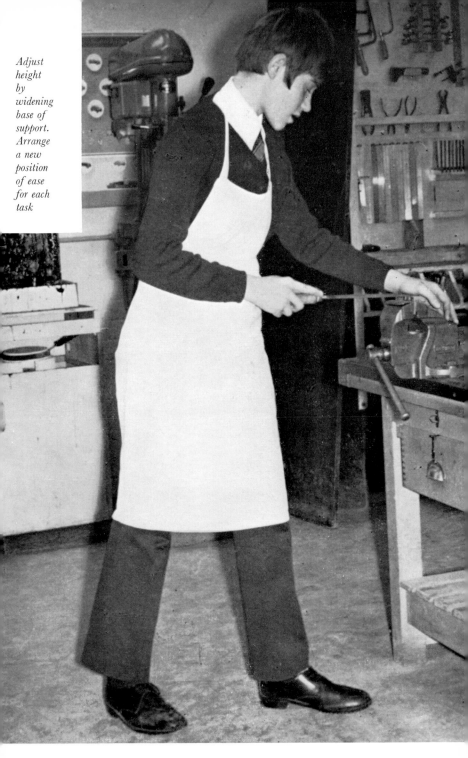

*Adjust
height
by
widening
base of
support.
Arrange
a new
position
of ease
for each
task*

PLATE 20
Working at the bench

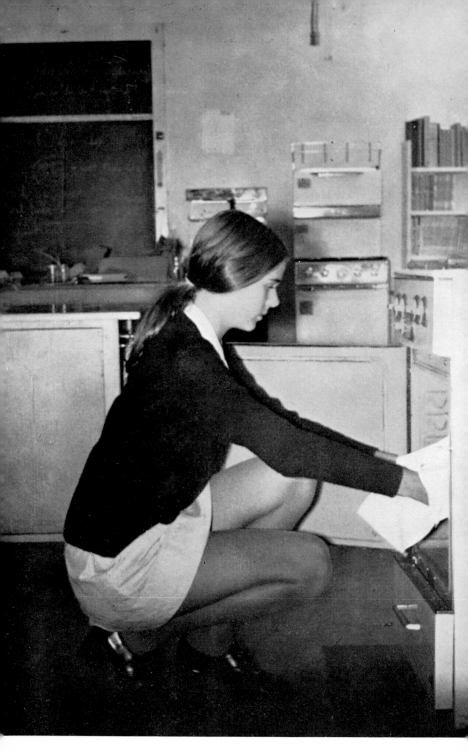

PLATE 21(a)
Working at the oven: the expanded habit, a position of ease

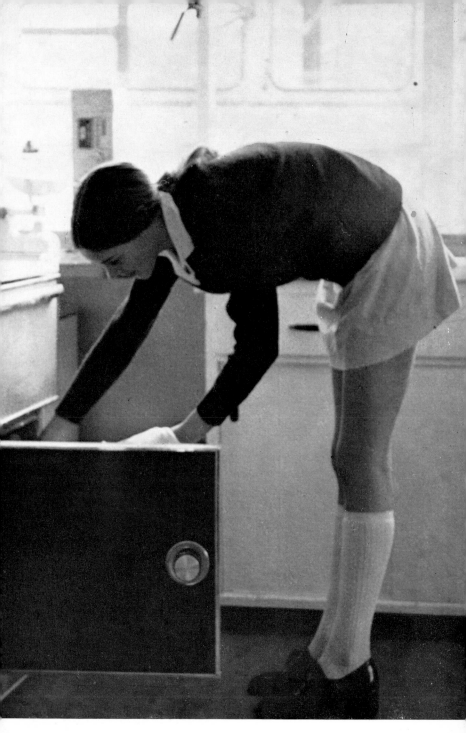

PLATE 21 (*b*)
Working at the oven: unnecessary tension, a position of strain

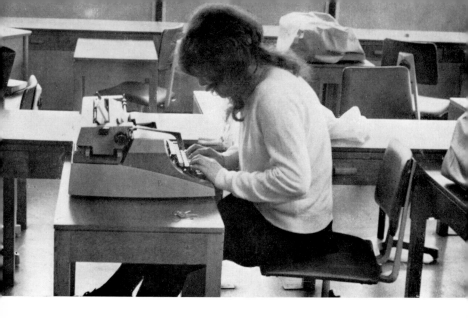

PLATE 22(*a*)—ABOVE
*Unnecessary tension and strain
can lead to pain in the
neck, back and wrists*

PLATES 22(*a*) AND 22(*b*)
Typing

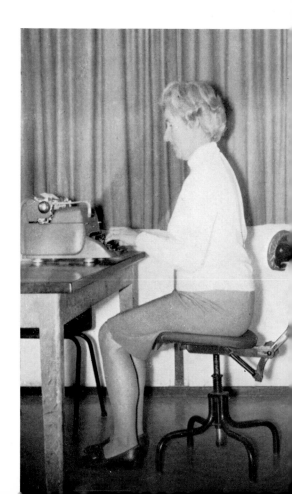

PLATE 22(*b*)
*Expanded habit, a position
of ease*

and games the aim should be to help young people to become more efficient in physical skills, to avoid fatigue, to remove muscular strain and to prevent the development of postural defects. To achieve this aim young people have to learn how to disperse the unnecessary muscular tension which causes wasteful activity. They have to learn to develop just enough muscular tone for the job in hand, and they have to learn how to maintain this stress-free, balanced posture until it becomes habitual in action. The suggestions which follow will help young people to achieve good use and sound mechanical mobility.

Teaching Sensory Appreciation

The classroom teaching of posture should begin with very simple anatomy. In this way, through drawing or modelling and through seeing, handling and discussing simple anatomical models, the children gain an appreciation of their own structure and bodily mechanics.

It is surprising how very few children have ever seen themselves full-length in a mirror, a valuable aid for checking how one moves (*see* p. 60).

The class teacher's attitude is very important, for good teaching in this subject, as in any other, evokes all the latent wonder and interest of the children. It is important to remember that the knowledge imparted is more than simply intellectual, for it involves *sensory* appreciation. For example, the children's attention may be guided to where the head balances at the top of the vertebral column. When this is identified as roughly between the ears, they can explore the movements of the head which are possible there at the top, watch each other's movements and then see the position of the joint in a skeletal model. This appreciation is an exceedingly important one, since many children and adults limit the freedom of this joint by a muscular tension of which they are unaware, a habit which causes headaches and similar pains.

Children enjoy finding out how the various parts of the body are constructed and what they can do in action, and by deliberately tensing and then relaxing their own arms and

E

hands they can be taught to differentiate between tenseness and relaxation. In this way they gain a vocabulary of words closely associated with the experience to which they refer which helps the teacher of physical education to give instruction in posture and also the children to observe movement around them.

In ordinary lessons the teacher also wittingly or unwittingly educates his pupils' physique, for by taking no notice of bad sitting, standing or writing positions he allows faulty habits to become conditioned which verbal advice alone cannot then correct.

Teaching Body Mechanics

Children should be shown good and bad movements and these can be timed with a stopwatch to prove strain or ease. Domestic movements should be introduced incidently at appropriate moments during primary and secondary school life. Many occupational movements should be demonstrated in the secondary school especially as a necessary preventative measure. For example, *standing* with the head forward (a position of strain involving the principle of more lean, more work) or with head erect (a position of ease which keeps the parts of the body as close to the vertical axis as possible).

Movement or Position	Principle involved
Head forward or erect	The more lean, the more work
Arm held midway-upward (position of strain	
Arm held horizontal (position of strain)	
Arm held midway-downward (position of ease)	
Arm held by side (position of ease)	Keep parts of the body as close to vertical axis as possible.
Forearm, elbows held *out*, forearms up or level (position of strain)	
Forearm, elbows held *in*, forearms up or level (position of ease)	

Many everyday occupational examples of these positions can easily be observed when young people are standing or sitting at desks, lathes, benches, counters, sinks, sewing machines, typewriters etc. (*see* Plates 19, 20, 21 and 22). Investigation has shown that over 80 per cent of young people do stand at their work for the greater part of the day (*see* Fig. 4 and p. 26).

Other examples of daily movements and positions with the principles of mechanics involved, which children should try out for themselves, are tabulated below.

These positions of the arms and forearms are used, for example, when sawing, filing, lifting, screwing and carrying (*see* Plate 20 and Fig. 8). Arrange the height of the body, by standing on a stool or steps, or kneeling, or by standing with feet astride to widen the base of support and lower the centre of gravity, so that the arms remain, as far as possible in a position of ease. In all activities children should be taught to keep the elbows in to the sides and when carrying a tray for example, to spread the fingers out underneath the tray, rather than hold the edges with the tips of the fingers.

Movement or position	*Principle involved*
Standing with the trunk slightly forward (strain)	The more lean, the more work
Standing with the trunk horizontal (strain)	
Squat (knee strain)	Keep parts of the body as close to vertical axis as possible.
Kneel (ease)	
Trunk bending downward with slight knee bending (ease)	
Trunk bending with a wide base of support (stability)	

These positions of the back are used when planing (*see* Plate 20 and Fig. 8—the children should turn sideways, open the legs to widen the base of support and lower the centre of gravity so that height is adjusted to the bench without stooping and the back is kept straight), filing and sawing. Planting, sowing seeds, choosing a book from a low library shelf, working at the oven (*see* Plate 21 and **Fig.** 8) are examples of movements which should be performed from the position of ease.

Lifting from table level	*Principles involved*
Standing with trunk slightly forward, feet together. Lifting using the *arms* (strain)	Stand close Use the largest, strongest muscle group and the greatest number of muscles
Standing with trunk slightly forward, feet together. Lifting using the *trunk* (strain)	Lower the centre of gravity over a wide supporting base
Standing with one leg slightly forward. Bend knees. Lifting using the *legs* (ease)	To lift heavy object when standing alongside it, advance the arm and leg forward on the same side and opposite the object
Lifting from the floor Lifting using the *trunk* (strain)	Lift close to the body Keep your equilibrium with a wide base of support
Lifting using *legs*, feet together (poor balance)	Use the mechanical advantage of bracing, *e.g.* lifting P.E. mats
Lifting using *legs*. One foot forward, over weight (good balance)	Use gravity to assist
	Momentum. Get a start

Improving Kinaesthetic Sense

The poise and efficiency of the teacher, his composure and easy, open attitude may well have an excellent effect upon his class as a whole. Everyone has heard the saying: "a noisy teacher, a noisy class;" so, too, a disturbed teacher, a disturbed class.

In his work teacher or child should make a habit of keeping his body and limbs in action, as *close to the vertical* as is convenient. There are scores of actions which need little energy in themselves, but which have to be done many times a day. If these actions are performed the easiest way, accumulated energy is saved and teacher or child will be fresher at the end of the day. So it is important to bring the watch or the book towards the eyes and not vice versa. A teacher looking at a seated child's work should *bend at the hips and knees* and not at the top of the back. *The more he leans, the more he works*: that is the guiding principle.

If the eyes alone will do, then use the eyes. If a head movement only will suffice, then use only a head movement. If a teacher is going to write on the blackboard he should only raise his arm and his hand (*see* Plate 24). There is no need to lean back, contract or raise the shoulders, or raise the head. It is the blackboard that should be raised or lowered, if possible.

There are, of course, numerous ways in which children can be shown how to improve their bodily movements during normal school activities.

Teachers are indebted to neurologists and psychologists for the scientific support which their investigations have given to changes in teaching techniques. Such changes in postural re-education are supported by the principle that thinking influences muscle action, either beneficially or detrimentally.

Its detrimental influence is well known to anyone who by continuing his day's work after going to bed at night produces a greater strain in his body instead of releasing it. As we have seen before, *the thought of an action is sufficient to ennervate the muscles which habitually perform it.*

Change is brought about by the conscious elimination of any faulty habit—verbal instruction alone is insufficient to bring about change. A young man with round shoulders had been given verbal instruction for twelve months in a training college about the need to avoid head retraction. In spite of this, by the end of the course he had still not learned to break his instinctive habit.

F. M. Alexander discovered that the body's sensory system seldom gives accurate information as to the position of the body in space or the inter-relationship of its parts. He realised the importance of what is known as the *kinaesthetic sense*, which enables people to perceive muscular motion, weight and position.[17]

In everyday life people who spontaneously prefer the better way of doing things are those who have the capacity to detect small differences of sensation. When the proper erect position is held, they not only sense the smallest change so that when necessary correcting their position is started quickly, but the

body also becomes capable of righting itself immediately
without preparation.

Some people, however, have no means of sensing the difference. Unless they are shown and experience the new sensation,
they never know about it at all. Constant training brings about
a better way of performing an activity, especially when the
person who is teaching the pupil has a fine kinaesthetic sense,
but generally speaking, without this teaching, it has been found
that a poor kinaesthetic sense gets poorer and a good one
better through habit.

Let the teacher ask his class to stand with their eyes closed
and to raise their arms exactly level with their shoulders. How
many will have their arms at different heights? (*See* Plate 23.)

In good posture the body is in balance, with no uneven
pressure between any of its joint surfaces. This posture can be
maintained in all positions or while making any movement
which is structurally possible, so long as there is no loss of
integrity in the vital neck, head and spine relationship. If
undue tensing of muscles impairs the freedom of this jointed
column, there will be a disturbance of co-ordination throughout
the body. If, for example, the pupil has the habit of compressing
his neck, causing his head to rest heavily on the spine, this
muscular pattern will influence every major movement he
makes.

In order to change this habit he must first become aware of
the pattern, refuse to follow it, and finally, redirect his movement
without disturbing the balance of the vertebral column. He
must stop and wait so that the new and better reaction may be
substituted for the old and faulty one. The greater the pupil's
ability to do this, the more rapid his progress will be.

Based on sound educational, sociological and psychological
principles, this method of helping the pupil to gain sensory
experience is fundamental and makes the changing of habit a
practical possibility. It is made possible above all by the
inhibitory pause, which serves to wipe clean the slate of habit.

Using a Mirror to Check Movement

This practice, which has been used by dancers for many
years, has not been used very much as a means of improving

techniques in physical education. Because so many children literally do not know how they use their bodies and have seldom (if ever) seen themselves full-length in a mirror they are not aware of the way they move. Because of habit, what they do feels right, though it is not necessarily so.

When faulty movements have been pointed out and a new use appreciated and "felt," then observation in a mirror can be a most valuable self-corrective. One little girl, for example, was most surprised to find when watching herself in a mirror, that when she stepped up on to a box, she raised and hunched her shoulders, rounded her back, compressed her head and did a number of movements with her arms.

CHAPTER 6

Teaching Good Habit in Schools—II

Woodhatch School

During a six-months' project on posture at Woodhatch (*see* also pp. 51–56) it was decided to give individual attention to certain children with marked postural difficulties, including four boys with poor co-ordination and asthma, an older boy (a stammerer) with remarkable over-tenseness throughout his body, and a very awkward and dreamy girl who had an unusually hollow back.

By direct observation and by means of film and tape recordings the teachers at Woodhatch accustomed themselves to noticing the children's "use" of their bodies in ordinary class activities, and they were surprised at the "normality" of over-tenseness. They soon realised that the core of the teaching problem in posture was that the muscles and joints of the body can grossly deceive their owner; what feels right is not necessarily right at all and in the long run might even be harmful. They found that it is not enough to ask a pupil to "set" the muscles of his arm and, having appreciated that as tense, to let them go and appreciate the difference. If the child is going to gain proficiency in movement he must be given experience of how and when he himself brings more effort to bear on a task than it requires. An example of this can be seen when a pupil, immediately on picking up his pencil to write, pulls in the joint surfaces of his hand, wrist and arm in such a way as to impair his performance and powers of attention. Yet he is quite unaware of this habit; and postural teaching, if it is going to be effective, must have constant reference to the habits and responses of boys and girls in real situations.

The objection may be raised that such a personal and individual form of teaching is not possible in a primary school. Yet the primary school is the most appropriate place to begin this study. That is why it is worth recalling how it was done at

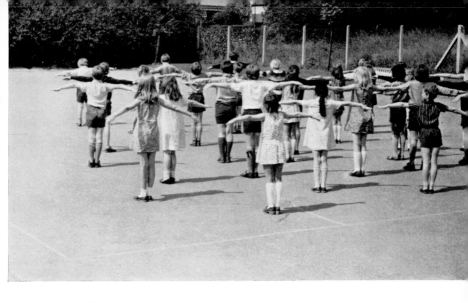

PLATE 23(a)
In the infants school

PLATES 23(a) AND 23(b)
At the verbal instruction:
"Arms level with
shoulders . . . raise!"
the results show
poor kinaesthetic sense

PLATE 23(b)
In the secondary
school

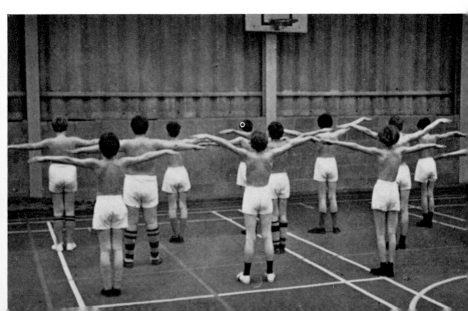

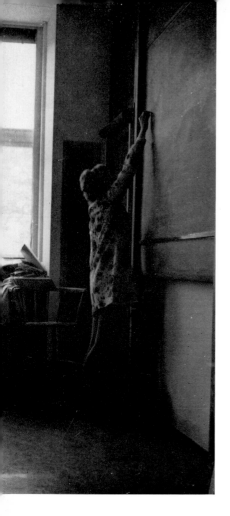

PLATES 24(*a*) AND 24(*b*)
Working at the blackboard

PLATE 24(*a*)
A position of strain

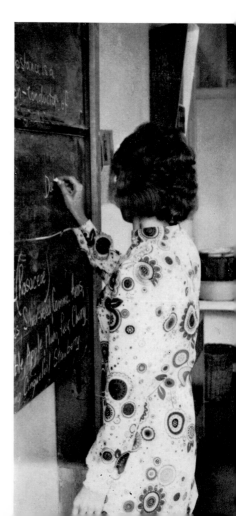

PLATE 24(*b*)
A position of ease

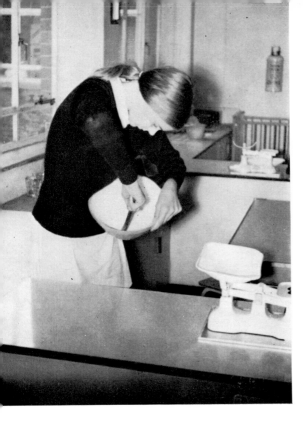

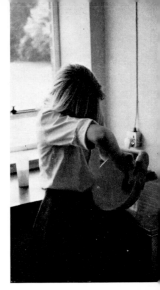

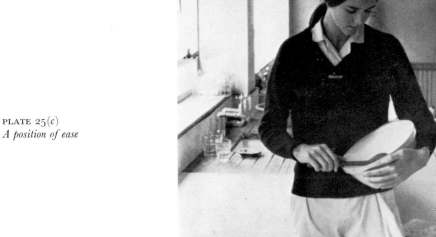

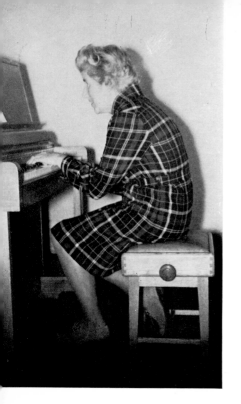

PLATE 26(*a*)
A contracted posture, a position of strain. Adjust height and position of stool— allow the spine to lengthen

PLATES 26(*a*) AND 26(*b*)
At the piano

PLATE 26(*b*)
The expanded posture, a position of ease

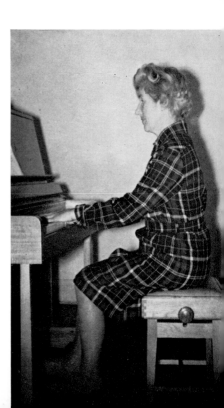

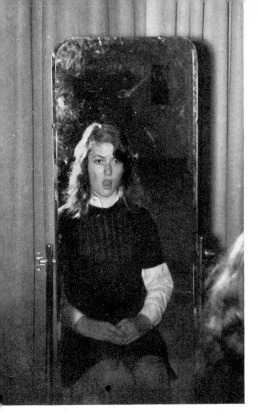

PLATES 27(a) AND 27(b)
Checking breathing using the mirror, saying the whispered "Aaagh"

PLATE 27(a)—LEFT

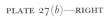
PLATE 27(b)—RIGHT

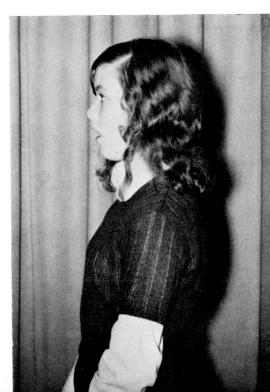

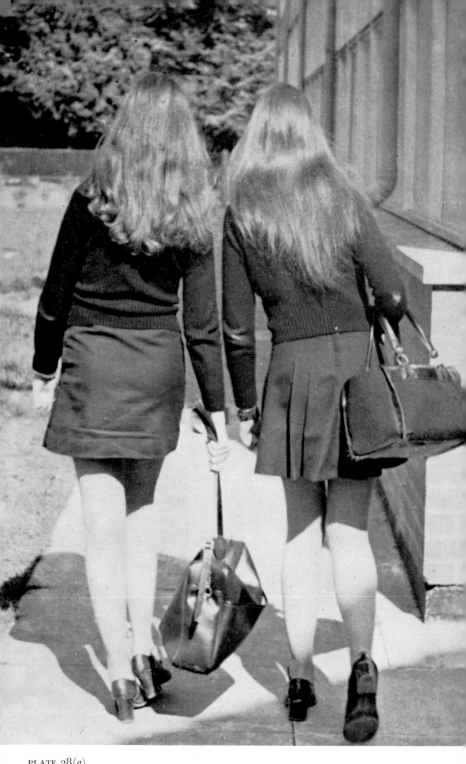

PLATE 28(a)
Walking and carrying a bag, showing poor use

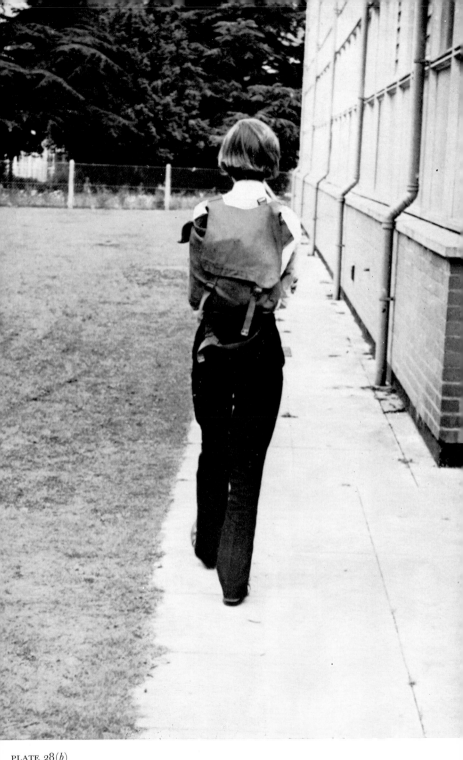

PLATE 28(b)
Walking and carrying a bag, with improved use

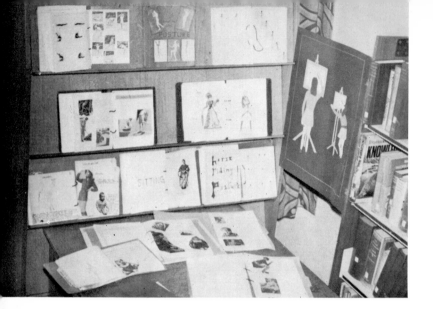

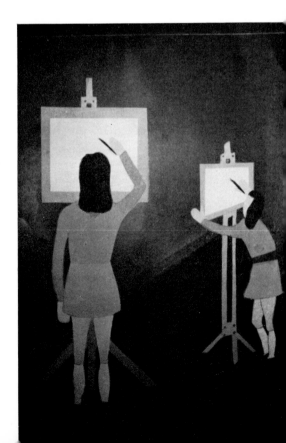

Woodhatch, where during the normal P.E. lesson five or six children (one group of several engaged in activities about the hall or field) were given specific instruction in a simple point of body mechanics. For example, one teacher decided to teach the children about the movement at the hip joint and show them the "closing the lid of the box" action in leaning forward while sitting. He then demonstrated distortions of this simple movement which involve the body in unnecessary strain.

Encouraging the children in his group to suggest what was at fault he found them doing so with enjoyment and interest. Asking one or two of them to demonstrate right and wrong ways he found them highly inventive in suggesting wrong ways. Throughout the fun they were having they were becoming increasingly aware that there was a *choice* in the way they could use their bodies. It was found that during the children's attempts to demonstrate right ways the crucial teaching point could be communicated easily, especially in teaching a small group. For example, when a child was asked to show the "right way" of performing a movement or holding a position he often did so quite unaware that his body was distorted through over-tenseness. Yet the rest of the group spotted it at once. Naturally the existence of this over-tenseness comes as a surprise to the child and this is a necessary experience. (*See Moving and Growing*, H.M.S.O., pp. 46–7.)

The teacher then showed the child how he could proceed in the right way without disturbing the stress-free arrangement of his body. The other children could see the difference so that if, as was not uncommon, the child said it did not "feel right," they could underline the teacher's assurance. This kind of personal experience made the children more observant when others were being taught; and after several repetitions of this kind of experience a "questing" state of mind was developed regarding the complete reliability of sensation. This was evident in each child's growing receptivity to instruction, his keenness to see his movement in the gymnasium mirrors, and his seeking corroboration from the teacher as an accepted necessity. Once this questing attitude was roused, teaching became a much simpler matter.

That much in posture is acquired by *deliberate and subconscious imitation* was clearly evident in the group and class teaching at

Woodhatch, for even children who received little or no tuition showed an improvement in postural habits, which could only have been acquired by some sort of imitation.

Tenseness has been described as the effort or activity unnecessary to the task in hand, and when a child comes to rest he should let go any effort which is not needed. Unfortunately, some children have lost this ability to come to rest, and this was specially noticeable in the children who were given individual attention at this school, although it was a common feature of children's behaviour generally. It has already been described how a child can be encouraged to have a moment of "stop" before jumping or vaulting, and it is well to remember that it is not sufficient for the teacher simply to give the instruction to do so, for most children have to learn for themselves how to come to rest, "to collect themselves" and to form a clear intention of what they are to do next.

It was found that this simple practice had a salutary effect upon the children's performance, enabling them, by shedding distraction and over-eagerness, to appreciate more steadily and attentively what was required of them in physical education.

Improvement in posture and movement and the achievement of habitual poise depend upon the growth and depth of the ability to "check-over." As this increases, so does the child's receptivity and it was found that the children who received postural training at Woodhatch improved also in their class-work, no doubt through their greater ability to pay attention. To the children who were given individual attention at this school, coming to rest was a burdensome task and their speed in gaining in proficiency in it varied greatly from child to child.

One boy with a history of asthma kept up his restless fidgetings for all but a few of the fifteen minutes of his first lessons, and he only gradually gained an awareness of his body while listening to instructions. Yet, after only a few weeks of postural education, he showed an easier manner and a much sunnier disposition, although his faulty habits of posture and movement showed only moderate change.

This is not unusual with those who have the over-tension habits associated with asthma, for the asthmatic violates flagrantly the principles of good use: the head is pulled back and down, the chest is made rigid, the back is hollowed, and air is forcibly sucked in. What is more significant is that the asthmatic's habit of breathing is always faulty, even at times when there are no obvious signs of asthma. A considerable period of postural education is often necessary radically to alter such habits, and it is interesting to notice that when malposture and tense movements (particularly of the neck, head and thorax) have been attended to, mild asthmatic tendency quite frequently disappears.

The response of three other children who had asthmatic over-tenseness was similar to that of the boy mentioned above: they became easier and more confident, but were slow to alter their habits at all profoundly. One highly intelligent boy, who quickly grasped the procedure and observed posture in others, found to his astonishment that it was virtually impossible for him to refuse his characteristic responses to move, and it was only after quite a number of lessons that he could do so. Only then was it possible to move in the direction of improved habit.

Lessons in posture helped him to feel the great over-tenseness of his neck and throat, a characteristic of an asthmatic child. This discovery was of itself a great relief to him for when he found himself starting to wheeze on the football field, by stopping and "letting himself go" he helped himself considerably.

Two other children at Woodhatch—a hollow-backed girl and a stammering boy—were of different temperaments. The little girl had such a marked deviation from a balanced alignment to start with that she found the experience of better posture thoroughly unfamiliar and unwittingly resisted instruction quite strongly by resuming her customary stance even while she was being instructed. This, of course, was usual and to be expected, but gradually, as she watched the other children during group instruction and as she used the gymnasium mirror she appreciated that what she felt wrong could, in fact, be "right." From then on she learned avidly and with increasing enjoyment, as was evident in a film which was made at the school. Being a child of very moderate ability, she enjoyed illustrating points from her special instruction in the small groups. In this way, she gained confidence generally and the help she gave in small-group instruction was considerable.

The stammering boy in the same class had the impediment

of over-tenseness throughout his body, not only in his lips, tongue and jaw. His movements were ungainly, his attitude one of withdrawal and apparent surliness. This boy responded so quickly to instruction in posture that his mother came to the school to express gratitude for "the change that had been made in her boy." What she had noticed was a greater confidence—he would go on an errand without a note, and would romp the streets with other boys, something he had been lothe to do before. She had noticed these changes at home before there was any great change in the boy's larger habits of movement. He had appreciated quite soon that he could ease his own burden himself and so could cope better. For the first time it was possible to allow him to read at morning assembly and he did it excellently. Later on he was given the job of school librarian and did it well.

On returning from the Easter holidays—a break of about three weeks—his stammer returned, but it lessened when his postural education was re-started and the term proceeded. At the end of the term he was able to perform in front of the movie-camera with considerable ease and confidence and with the camera closely trained on him he chatted impromptu with a teacher who was virtually a stranger to him.

On the last day of the summer term when he was leaving the primary school he again took a major part in the closing assembly. On this occasion his mother was invited and came with other parents—he had not told her when he had read at Easter.

This boy's increasing self-confidence had helped him in many ways in addition to those already mentioned. He learned to ride a bicycle, something which he had said he would never do, and he enjoyed much more relaxed sleep instead of the frequent restless nights to which he had been accustomed. This boy has never stammered since that time.

One observation which is worth making on the experience gained at Woodhatch is that good posture is not necessarily allied to high intelligence or athletic physique. The children with fair posture were not all the same types, though the one thing they had in common was their readiness to have a go, to welcome and adapt new experience.

It was also evident that postural education can readily take its place in the curriculum and presents little or no administrative difficulty. Ideally, relaxation exercises should be taught in a moderately spacious room or hall which is quiet and warm, the children lying on their backs on the floor on some kind of rubber matting. But even in schools without such facilities— the work at Woodhatch was done in "prefabs"—a great deal can be done to improve body mechanics and general habits of use in pupils.

De Stafford School

A similar project was carried out in a large secondary school. The Alexander technique was introduced to over two hundred boys and girls in the second year aged twelve to thirteen years.

Experience gained in the primary school project was used and additional methods were tried. A specialist Alexander teacher also attended for two complete days each week. Talks were given to all members of staff first, to explain the aims and what was being attempted; these lecturettes were informative and illustrated by use of the epidiascope and film. As preparation, prior to the actual beginning of the experiment, all second year classes were given lessons, as part of their normal science course, on the skeletal and muscular systems of the body and the potential movements of the joints and limbs.

The project covered the second half of the spring term and the first half of the summer term, separated by a two- to three-week break at Easter.

An attempt was made to introduce this technique of education and re-education into school life without upsetting or altering the normal school timetable. Introductory talks with films of about twenty minutes were given to the children during assembly time on four occasions in the first week of the project. These explained how to recognise undue and unnecessary tension, the correct use of body mechanics and how to observe and recognise such postures—the main aims were to make pupils *aware* of the factors involved in acquiring and maintaining good use of the body; to *teach* body mechanics in all situations and to develop a class or *group approach* to this subject which is preventative as well as re-educational.

The project was important because poor posture and poor body mechanics lead to functional disorders, the consequence of which affect the receptivity of the body so that the learning processes are impaired. Economically, the national annual cost of such disorders and complaints adds up to many millions of lost working days and many millions of pounds.

The specialist teacher visited the pupils in their various rooms and school activities, getting them to realise that there was a choice in the manner in which one could perform. When filing in the metalwork room for example, in addition to being shown how to handle a file the pupil was shown how to arrange his body at the work bench to the best stress-free mechanical advantage (*see* Plates 12, 20, 21, 22 and 25 and Fig. 8). The same applied in the practical rooms for woodwork, cookery, needle-work, art, technical drawing, etc. The staff were most co-operative throughout, and the children appeared to be interested and to enjoy this additional application to their work.

A teacher stated:

"real progress has been made over the practical subjects. The girls have seen the point of it (the project) during cookery, as greater efficiency is obtained, with washing up, mixing ingredients, etc. (*see* Plate 25). In art both girls and boys are making pictures full of movement, this has shown real application backed by the excellent teaching of the art mistress where the understanding of a forward and upward direction of the spine is reflected in the work. On the other hand, however, progress is slow over class posture. The girls especially really do appear to find it hard to appreciate that it really does matter how they *sit* both in the classroom and at needlework.

The boys on the whole appear to sit in better postures. Regular practice is needed with plenty of practical demon-strations with desks and chairs, so that children of all sizes can adapt themselves to the furniture.

It is felt, however, that much of the beneficial work will be defeated if we do not tackle the problem of the heavy bags and cases that they carry around from class to class and back home each day. However well they move in school, and however much they think of upward release, the fast growing younger pupils will not be sufficiently strong, well grown, or stabilised, to combat the pull downwards and round, or the shoulder strain of the weight. The former method of carrying the satchel or rucksack distributing and balancing the weight on the back could still well be the best method" (*see* Plate 28).

All pupils were also asked to produce (in half a term) a folder project on this subject by collecting newspapers, magazine cuttings, etc., showing children and adults of all ages in varying positions, occupations and postures—adding relevant comments about the pictures. It was suggested that they collected postures of people in different countries and pictures from various periods in history; to find out and decide if environment affected good body management, if furniture did, and so on. Many pupils also produced large posters illustrating various activities performed in different rooms (*see* Plate 29). These were displayed as constant reminders of sound use. All the 200 folders and posters were made into an exhibition at the half-term stage and created considerable interest to the viewers, including many who had not been involved.

The visiting specialist teacher arranged to see some pupils with individual needs at fifteen-minute intervals during the lunchtime. One short, stocky girl of twelve years was suffering from headaches almost every night (this was discovered from the latest medical inspection at school). It was found that she held her head slightly to one side and she could only turn it a short distance to right or left. The cause of the headaches was great tension both of neck muscles and the corresponding muscles of the trunk. There was a knot of compression in the cervical vertebrae. Through the few minutes instruction twice a week her headaches became far fewer and her head looser and freer in turning. She learned to release the neck and turn her head to help avert the headaches, and after only seven short lessons was making rapid progress.

A tall girl of 5 feet 9 in. aged thirteen years had developed a pronounced stoop (noted at her medical inspection). After only nine short lessons, she needed only to be seen once a week because she had developed a good grasp of the principles of the technique and was able to help herself. Her back soon became much stronger.

At the end of the first half term the staff were asked to comment on a list of questions from their own observations. They agreed that with their limited experience of noticing unnecessary tension and malposture they could only note obvious or gross examples. It was significant, therefore, that the great majority observed "unnecessary tension" in children; about 70 per cent agreed that there was little correlation between intelligence and body management, over 50 per cent felt that "body management of children at school deteriorated with age." One teacher said that "a marked improvement was shown with conscious effort in the second year—but without this 'awareness' the answer would be deterioration" (rather than an improvement or constant performance). Of the factors affecting good or bad use, unsuitable furniture easily headed the list, with such causes as the carrying of heavy satchels and bags, sitting badly for a large part of the day, and boredom, also being mentioned by a number of staff. The answers to whether boys or girls showed better body mechanics or if it varied with age, were inconclusive and contained many qualifications.

Another teacher commented: "from my work with two forms in the second year it seems to me that the major advantage of the project is that it made the children *aware* of posture. Previously for them it did not exist."

In view of the previous comment it would seem to be necessary closely to follow up the present work with *constant reminders*—attention from the teacher in class to the various problems, *posters* around the school, occasional work on the subject in various lessons.

One interesting factor has been how the children have related the project to their lives outside the school. They refer to how their parents and brothers and sisters sit, how the work relatives did affects their posture, illnesses of neighbours caused by body management, etc.

Children thought that the project was particularly helpful when it aided them in practical terms, *e.g.* being taught the correct way to carry things.

Some boys suggested that startling posters on the lines of those used to discourage smoking would help.

The whole term's project therefore became a complete educational integrated study cutting across all departments and all aspects of school life.

Hints for Teachers

First, some points to bear in mind *during any type of class or school activity.*

1. Observe the child's body as a whole; especially notice the alignment of the head, neck and spine. Remind children to let the spine lengthen all the time.
2. Remember to visualise good *skeletal* relationships, and not be led astray by body contours, nor by aesthetic preference for a type of build.
3. Check the children sitting.
4. Check the children lifting or carrying.
5. Check the children standing, in the hall, playground or classroom.
6. Check breath-holding in children.
7. Learn to observe tenseness in children, for example:
    (*a*) In the face: pursing lips, frowning.
    (*b*) In the hand: pencil pressed too hard so that the work shows through a number of pages. Tight knuckles.
    (*c*) In the throat: harshness of the voice often indicates tenseness when talking or singing.
    (*d*) Jerky movements indicate tenseness.
    (*e*) Poor mechanical use or movement leads to tension.
    (*f*) Raised shoulders (the most common fault) consume energy unnecessarily, and so on.
8. Encourage children to check each other's *use*, in the same way as they check each other's reading, memory-work or sums.
9. Remember that imitation is a potent teacher, wittingly and unwittingly.
10. Miming activities can be included in many lessons, including drama, singing, dancing and music, when the

F

emphasis should be on efficient movement. The children can imagine that they are conducting an orchestra, playing the violin or flute, controlling the traffic, hitting with a hammer, searching for something on the floor, swinging a large hammer with two hands, and so on. Check the expanded state during each movement. Demonstrate with children showing good performances.

Second, some points to bear in mind *during the physical education lessons*: some of the points refer to technique and some to class organisation.

1. Stress and choose activities which encourage *joint separation*. For example, hanging and climbing movements correctly performed, rhythmical movements—these are useful for joint mobility—and loosening exercises. They are efficient and economical of energy. Skilled movements are more rhythmical than unskilled movements. Relaxation exercises (already described). Games such as volley ball, netball and basket ball which incorporate jumping and reaching movements.

2. Omit and avoid activities which compress the spine, or pull in the joint surfaces and limit or restrict movement; both are likely to cause damage. Burt (1958) pointed out that the approximation of joint-surfaces by muscle contraction is a factor in the pain of rheumatoid arthritis where faulty posture and muscular hypertension are combined.[18] In addition, osteo-arthritic changes may be produced by constant muscular misuse; when this is already present it may become painful under the strain of muscular tension.

   Compression movements to avoid are those that press the head backwards and many types of spanning exercise, which unless performed with good use, can do more harm than good. Weight lifting can be performed in a mechanically advantageous manner (bending at the hips and knees and keeping the back aligned, etc.) but creates harmful use if the head is compressed and the expanded "norm" disturbed in the lift.

   Observation of Covent Garden porters carrying

many baskets balanced on their heads showed that they almost without exception had good use. This was apparently survival of the fittest; those unable to carry out the job well had been eliminated.

3. Give the children practice in localising movements and so save energy.

4. Analyse movements you find are not being correctly carried out.

5. Make use of mirrors as a teaching aid.

6. Emphasise the pause or "stop" before a movement, *e.g.* a vault, a jump, etc., in order to "check-over" and get rid of superfluous muscular tension; then get the children to *choose* a new improved pattern of movement.

7. It is in the group practices that most *individual* attention can be paid to the pupil. Do not try to progress too quickly. It takes time to change habit, even in children. Do not try to do too many things at once. It is not necessary for every child to change round to every group activity in every lesson. It may take some weeks before they complete the circuit of activities. On the other hand, do not spend too long at any one time on one activity; the teacher must sense when the time is ripe to change to something else.

(*a*) Group children according to their physical abilities initially (this does not prevent them from being grouped according to games skill during some other part of the lesson).

(*b*) Some will have a number of faults, so treat the most pronounced faults first, *e.g.* habitually raised shoulders, poked-out chin, or head retraction.

(*c*) Teach one new activity to the class as a whole, for example "balance along a beam with alternate knee bending below the beam." Get the children to demonstrate. Indicate points to look for in the balance itself and in the body management during the performance (*e.g.*, keep the torso as upright as possible throughout the movement, keep the head, neck and spine aligned and released, let the shoulders hang loosely, not raised, elbows relaxed, good movement in all joints involved, eyes looking ahead, level not fixed or staring, and so on).

(*d*) Let the children go to their group corners and all practise the same activity as a group, under the supervision of a leader. The teacher then supervises each group in turn and gives individual tactile correction if necessary to each child in turn, in the same way as a teacher now corrects a child showing some gross position.

(*e*) Teach a second new practice to the whole class.

(*f*) Return to group corners. The teacher supervises the new practice with one group while the others practice their first activity.

(*g*) Move the groups around so that the teacher again sees each individual in turn performing the new activity.

(*h*) Gradually, depending upon progress, build up a separate practice for each group.

(*i*) Pay specific attention to the "group fault," *e.g.* the head retraction, during the performance of, say, the "balance with knee bending" activity. Notice how the head is drawn back and down, compressed when going down or coming up. Make sure that the children realise this—let the group observe and correct each other, with the teacher supervising.

8. Make the children conscious that you are watching their movements and use in activity all the time, *e.g.* when they are skipping, picking up a dropped ball, pushing or pulling, stepping through a hoop, etc. Give remarks to various members of the class: "don't bend your back John when you pick up the ball, but bend at the hips and knees. Let me see you pick up the ball again, now!" or, "Mary, keep your head still and let your shoulder drop when you are skipping. Now try it again, lightly and loosely."

9. Give instructions slowly and concisely. After a pause, to allow the children to start from "rest" and to form a clear intention of what they are going to do, make the final word indicate the manner of performance, *e.g.* fast, slow, tense, relaxed, heavy, light.

10. Give the children time to perform each movement before going on to the next instruction.

11. Remember, it is only after the verbal command has been

given that *you start teaching*. Quickly then, get around and among your class—some will need "putting right," as David did during his dance. Verbal instruction alone will correct few faults, because in so many children their kinaesthetic sense is faulty—they cannot "feel" if they are right or wrong, through lack of experience.

12. The teacher should always be in such a position that he can see the whole room, and have in mind which particular activity he is going to stress during the lesson; he should so arrange things that at the same time he can see what the other groups are doing, and be able to give an occasional hint to them to let them know that he is watching them.

13. There should be variety in the lesson, but there should not be continually new forms of exercise: it takes time to learn to feel an exercise.

14. The teacher should ask himself if the children have been kept active most of the time. Remember the type of work that has been discussed does not make for a slow, ponderous lesson. It adds extra interest and purpose for the children. The aim is to be relaxed in activity, whether it is a vigorous run or a slow balance.

15. The teacher should ask himself at the end of the lesson if there have been any "dead pauses." There should be pauses, with a purpose (*see* paragraph 6 above) for both teacher and children. But there should not be dead pauses, when nothing is being done, for example, waiting for the marking or apparatus to be arranged, or waiting for a turn at the apparatus, or because the children are not sure what to do. Unless there is a clear intention of what to do, performance will be poor.

CHAPTER 7

Checking our Use and Movement

Standing

When a child is standing correctly, his neck muscles will be released, not contracted or stretched. His head will be level, tilted neither backwards nor forwards. His shoulders will lie lightly, not braced, pulled forward or raised. His breathing will be easy with a gentle abdominal movement accompanying the movement of the chest. His pelvis will be level, neither tucked in nor stuck out. His legs will be straight without bracing the knees, and his weight will fall evenly over the feet. His spine, to achieve all these aims, must be upright, without being braced or stiff.

As this expanded state of posture is of such prime importance—the starting point and norm for all movement—it will be useful to discuss it in more detail.

Let the feet feel the support of the floor, let them spread, do not claw the toes. See that the weight of the body is equally distributed over both feet, forwards, backwards and sideways.

Attention should then be directed in turn to other parts of the body. Release the head and neck muscles and allow the spine to lengthen. Do not *try* to do this, do not *stretch* upward, do not *make* it lengthen: just allow it to do so. By trying to stretch, unnecessary tensions will be produced.

This feeling or releasing of the neck and head is fundamental to all efficient movement. It must be continually checked whether the body is stationary or moving and it can be done on all sorts of occasions: sitting in a bus, strap-hanging, shaving or reading. Children can check-over at the beginning or end of a lesson or whenever they are still for a short time, for example when the bell rings or the register is called.

Attention can be directed to a part of the body without actually thinking or doing anything about it. A teacher can be thinking about the history lesson he is giving to his class and, at the same time, be aware that Johnny is gazing out of the window.

In directing a child's attention to any part of the body where superfluous muscular activity should be released, the teacher may initially hold the area of tension, his grip indicating the direction in which the released tension is flowing.

In checking the fundamental standing position attention must be paid to the hips, knees and ankles. The shoulders should be freed and the arms hanging loosely like a yoke. The breathing should be released.

From this position—the norm—any movement or series of movements may start. In a vast range of activities, bending from the hip joint forms the primary movement.

Sitting

The most common act of all which demands the co-ordinated movements of hip and knee joints is that of *sitting down* on a chair from a standing position and rising again (*see* Fig. 9). Anyone who can do this well will have solved most bending problems, and the way of doing it well depends on maintaining the easy expanded state of the torso and bending the hip and knee joints with no curving of the back.

First sit on a flat-bottomed chair or stool which should only be high enough to permit the feet to be flat on the floor without any undue pressure on the thighs. Check the sitting posture, feel the support of the chair, let the hands lie lightly in the lap. See that there is no tension in the legs and the buttocks and that the neck is free. Check the head to see that it is properly balanced, and the whole body, the whole torso, should be easily upright without stretching, without slumping (*see* Plate 9). The shoulders should be lying lightly, neither braced nor dropped. If this has been done properly the body will have achieved an easy expanded state.

Now experiment a bit. Lean forward until the elbows rest on the knees. Do it without curving the back. Move *entirely* from the hip joints, yet with no feeling of rigidity in the back. Move backward and lean forward like this a number of times. Look down leaning forward, bringing the glance level in the upright position.

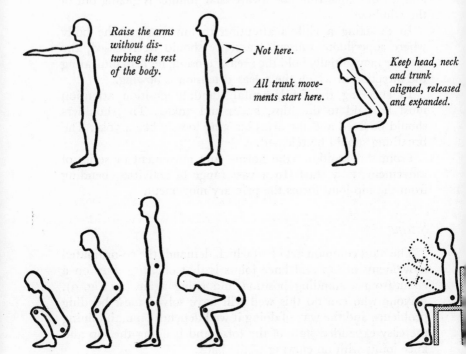

Raise the arms without disturbing the rest of the body.

Not here.

All trunk movements start here.

Keep head, neck and trunk aligned, released and expanded.

(a) *A great many movements originate at the hip joint, e.g. sitting, picking up, lifting.*

(b) *The main hinges for bending, at the ankle, knee and hip joint, should be used without compressing the spine.*

FIG. 9—*Let the spine lengthen.*

It would be helpful to mime a number of actions that are performed in a sitting position, for example, bending down to tie a shoelace, playing the piano or typing (*see* Plates 22 and 26) —how many people get a pain in the back or neck! Check all movements in a mirror or work in pairs and check one another.

These hip movements can be done without a chair, by going down to a deep squat position with both feet flat on the floor. This needs practice with adults, but it does utilise the ankle, knee and hip joints very well.

Notice how the very young children play on the beach with their buckets and spades (*see* Plate 2). It is a very natural position, but with modern furniture people get out of the habit of using these joints fully. It is worth remembering that over one-quarter of the world's population still sits in this deep squat position.

Walking

When you think of *walking*, you usually think of the feet, but the primary control of walking lies in the balance of the head, the tension of the neck muscles and the position of the spine (*see* Plate 8). Start from the standing position, previously explained—the expanded state of posture. Stand in front of a mirror. Have a chair each side of you, the backs of the chairs turned in towards you. Check your general posture in this way. Make sure your weight is evenly balanced over both feet, and over the whole surface of the feet. Your weight should not fall chiefly on the inner or the outer edges of the feet, nor heavily on the heels or the toes. The toes pointing straight ahead should be released and nearly flat—not curled underneath the foot.

Support yourself by touching the backs of both chairs with the tips of your fingers, but don't press down. Raise one knee till the thigh is almost parallel with the floor, the lower part of the leg hanging freely, ankle free and toes dropped. The important thing is not to lean heavily over to the side. There should be hardly any movement sideways.

Now lower the foot slowly—don't drop it or put it down heavily. The toes will touch the floor first if the ankle is free—though in quick walking, of course, the heel touches the ground first. If you carry out these instructions properly, the foot will land almost its own length in front of the other. Repeat this movement several times with each leg alternately.

Don't look down at your feet. Look straight ahead. Sense the movement of the hip, knee and ankle. When you have done this several times, dispense with the chairs.

When you have done this broken-up walking for some time, gradually take quicker steps. But still continue to sense the balance of your body, the movement of each joint, the way your feet touch the floor. See that the feet point straight ahead

G

and are turned neither inwards nor outwards. The body should not bob up and down or sway from side to side. A relaxed gentle arm swing can assist locomotion, but care should be taken not to disturb the expanded torso by raising the shoulders or by giving the appearance of levering the body along by the arms. Walking can be pleasure. It is certainly one of our best forms of exercise, but bad posture can make it an ordeal.

This analysis of the movements of the body produces an awareness of the way the body may be used as an instrument. By choosing the essentials of sitting and standing, etc. and by showing the action and making it simple and formal, it is possible to bring out the details of habitual movement.

To become aware of how things are done is almost all that is needed to bring about a change. If, for instance, a child has a tendency to pull his head back on to his spine whenever he rises or lifts something, almost all he needs to do to change this habit is to notice the fact more and more: sensing it and seeing it in a mirror. The more his appreciation of the habit grows, the more it tends to disappear, hence the value of short practices which "enlarge" the movements of the body. By such practice new and better habits can be established by day-to-day informal use. In time, they become as natural as the previous ones were.

Breathing

Breathing is the next thing to notice. First, re-check posture whether sitting or standing. Then, without pulling back the head or raising the shoulders, open the mouth and say "Aaaaaah!" in a prolonged whisper. This should be done without taking a deep breath and without squeezing the last drop of air out. . . . Keep comfortably within the ordinary range of breathing (*see* Plate 27).

As "Aaaaaah!" is being said, the gentle contraction of the abdomen should be sensed. Now close the mouth and allow the chest to fill again. Do not take a great gulp of air, just let the chest fill easily. Pause for a moment or two allowing the breath to come and go gently, then say "Aaaaaah!" again, and so on. Regard this not as a breathing exercise in the ordinary sense of the word, but rather as a breathing examination—to ensure that the breathing movements are not being restricted.

The making of the "Aaaaaah!" sound—an open-throated vowel sound—may be described as an enlargement of breathing. Do it with a mirror. Some children, just before opening their lips, tip their heads back a bit and fix the neck. A few will notice this from the mirror, or from being told about it, or even from the quality of the "Aaaaaah!" sound. If the throat is tight, the sound will be a little harsh.

Some children, on the other hand, are surprised to discover that they cannot let their jaws drop. (The hinge is just in front of the ears.) This is because they usually have the jaw rather tight and to let it go or even ease it "feels all wrong." If it does feel wrong, they should experiment in front of a mirror. They will find it looks all right especially if they "think a smile" just before letting go. (They may never have thought of a smile as an easing of the muscles of expression.) They should notice, too, that the tongue lies at rest on the floor of the mouth, the tip almost touches the back of the lower teeth.

Children should practise this whispered "Aaaaaah!" sound several times until they are sure of the sequence. When they have made use of it to help them to notice how they breathe, they should then use it as they practise movement and lifts. Many children hold their breath when lifting; it is unwise to do so and it is a strain.

Breath-holding also goes with anxiety, and there are times when children are anxious with good reason. There are other times when they are unreasonably or unduly anxious. A child who has accustomed himself to being aware of his body and how he uses it, realises that he can shed his burden of undue anxiety when he releases unnecessary tension and, in particular, allows his breathing to flow undisturbed.

As he becomes proficient in maintaining an expanded state of posture in activity he will notice that he is less troubled by little things and that there is an improvement in his poise and composure. By slowing down and analysing his own movements a teacher will notice when the stress-free arrangement of his own body is disturbed. He will find that it is easier to locate any habit which is contributing to backache or muscular strain, and that it is easier to learn to alter a habit or movement in slow motion.

It is not suggested that a teacher and his class should move like Chinese mandarins or sit primly away from the chair back. But once a teacher or a child has learned how to maintain the expanded state of posture and become accustomed to appreciating their balance and surroundings while they are moving and acting, the transition to applying what they have learned to normal activities, at normal speeds, and then to difficult lifts or difficult situations of any kind, is simpler than if they tried to cope with everything at one and the same time.

Once they have learned to take sound posture into simple and formal movements both teacher and child can learn to take it into informal and even casual movements with attendant poise and efficiency.

The Rules of Sound Movement

1. Standing holding the weight in front of the body.
   (a) Widen the base of support to make balance easier.
   (b) Relax elbows to the side.
   (c) Hold bulk of the weight close to the body.
   (d) Grip with the entire hand instead of the clenched fist.
2. Never hold a forward bent position for long periods when the same result may be accomplished in the erect position.
3. When it is necessary to bend forward, place one leg forward (it adds stability, extends the base of support, and acts as a prop to give greater balance).
4. Whenever required to maintain a lower working level for a period of time (e.g. on the floor, library shelf, with pets), squat or kneel so that as nearly as possible the body weight may be kept upright over the base of support (see Plate 21(a) and Fig. 8).
5. Keep the centre of gravity moving and behind you when moving an object by pulling. For example, do not hold the body weight rigid when pulling, but distribute the body weight from the forward to the rear leg by rocking backward while pulling.
6. Never lift a heavy weight upward and off its supporting

surface when you can slide it with its weight remaining on its supporting surface.

7. Relax muscles where you can; contract muscles hard only when you must.

8. Use the largest possible muscle groups and the largest number of muscles.

Localising Movement

Teach simple movements without disturbing the expanded torso. This is fundamental: it implies conservation of energy and an absence of strain. Ask any group of standing children to raise their arms forward and it will be noticed that a number lean backward at the same time as they raise their arms.

Ask for a pencil to be picked up ready for writing and often it will be seen that the fingers are contracted and the joint surfaces drawn together restricting movement (*see* Plate 11); the pencil is lifted in a vice-like grip, shoulders are raised and one elbow planted firmly on the desk. Try to limit the amount of effort and the work done for a simple movement. Father will find that he can release much of his grip on the screwdriver or saw and still get the desired result. The car driver can release much of his grip on the steering wheel and still maintain complete control of his direction.

Teachers can help children to prevent the backward movement of the trunk when raising the arms forward if they get the children to *lie down*. Then, with the back supported, the children can raise first one, and then two arms without disturbing the rest of the body. Get them to practise this with the least effort. If the back tends to become hollowed in this position, then to prevent it, the teacher should get the children to raise the knees and keep the feet flat on the floor—some support can be placed under the knees if necessary.

Progress to *kneeling* and then raise one and two arms forward —add other simple movements of the arms without disturbance. For example, conduct an orchestra, play the violin, control the traffic in mime, without affecting the expanded state of the torso.

Finally, get the children to stand and repeat arm movements.

Mime underarm quoit or ball throwing with a follow-through in the same stress-free manner.

Analyse other simple movements such as "picking up something" or "writing." Perform each stage in slow motion and check the expanded norm, also check each return movement. Repeat and repeat until the *correct* performance becomes habitual. The teacher must continually remind the children to let the spine ease and lengthen at all times. *Make haste slowly—* new habits require time and constant correct repetition. When the activity can be done efficiently then normal speed can be introduced.

Here is an example of analysing the movement involved in "picking up an object" from the floor.

1. Stand with the feet slightly astride (check the expanded posture).
2. Bend the knees forward and let the arms dangle (check again to see that there was no disturbance during this movement). Stretch again without altering the norm (check).
3. Lower the trunk forward slightly at the same time, until the fingertips lightly touch the knees; a gorilla-like position. (This is a good position for checking the released head and neck alignment of the back, etc.) Return to the standing position (check).
4. Repeat 3 again and pick up an object from the floor. Remember to allow the trunk to lengthen all the time. Do not reach too far; have the object about one foot in front of the toes (check the released torso in that position). Return to the standing position (check).
5. Repeat as in 4—then add turning the head left and right in "picking up" position.
6. Stand with one foot slightly forward and perform the same movement, *i.e.* like a curtsy (check the norm when down and on return).
7. Walk, stop and pick up an object, then straighten up and continue walking.

Here is another example, the "writing" movement analysed.

1. Check the sitting position, as already described.

2. Lean the trunk forward slightly from the sitting position and let the arms dangle (check). Return to the upright sitting position (check the released, expanded torso).
3. Still sitting, raise one elbow slightly forward and outward (check the norm—especially that the shoulder is not raised nor tense). Move the arm in various directions (check).
4. Lean slightly forward and rest one forearm on the desk (check the head, neck and shoulders. See that the buttocks are well-supported and not raised off the seat etc.).
5. Hold a pencil loosely between the thumb and first two fingers and then make patterns in the air, moving only the fingers and wrist (check head, neck, spine, shoulders, breathing, arm, wrist, fingers, etc., for unnecessary tension).
6. Combine the movements above and write something on the paper. Start and end by checking the expanded state of posture. While acquiring the correct performance of any movement the child must be like a juggler. He must start by checking the whole body for release—the norm—and then with that as a starting point *add to it* (not forget about it and start something new, but add to it, while keeping a check on the norm, any other movement he wishes).

These progressive stages would naturally be introduced gradually into lessons and the rate of progress would depend upon the individual children, as in all learning.

Checking One Another

This applies not only to the everyday and occupational activities which have been described already, but also to games and sports practices. Children quickly appreciate right and wrong use once it has been pointed out to them, and they can check all sorts of movements, *e.g.* landing from a height, throwing and catching, balancing, climbing and running. It is interesting to notice that quite often a child can be seen running with his head pulled back and even leaning backwards. From a distance he looks as if he is being held back by some invisible force and could go much faster if released, which indeed he could (*see* Plate 17).

CHAPTER 8

Conclusions

One hundred years ago the great Nonconformist philosopher and educationalist, Herbert Spencer, felt strongly that "the competition of modern life" was so keen that few people could bear it without injury. "Already," he reflected in his famous book on education "thousands break down under the high pressure they are subject to. If this pressure continues to increase, as it seems likely to do, it will try severely even the soundest constitutions. Hence it is becoming of especial importance that the training of children should be carried on as not only to fit them mentally for the struggle before them, but also to make them physically fit to bear its excessive wear and tear."[19]

Today, observes a social historian of the first half of the twentieth century, we are a healthier nation in every respect except one—our nerves. "The wear and tear of modern life, the increased tempo and the gnawing of anxiety are telling on us. This is a major problem of modern industrial societies in general, not a peculiarity of Britain. Neuroses and bodily illnesses that have a pronounced psychological side to them, such as duodenal ulcers, are a growing problem." So, too, is the increasing incidence of coronary disease, one of the causes of which is now recognised in stress and tension. "We need to learn more about the principles of all-round health, psychological and physical, in an industrial community."[20]

Many personnel and welfare officers are already doing a great deal to encourage this scientific approach to health, by attempting to reduce the increasing physical tensions evident in their workers. It has been an aim of this book to show that "there is an intimate relationship between anxiety and muscular tension"[21] and that by reversing the process and relaxing the tension the adult or the child can be relieved of pain and anxiety. Evidence had shown that a significant proportion of children and young people were physically not at their best and that the misuse of the body in various ways was the commonplace rather than the exception. Continued into adult life this bodily mismanagement is revealed in irritating, painful and, often, expensive complaints which, although they are regarded as the penalties of growing old, could well have been prevented or ameliorated in childhood.

At the present time it is apparent from reports, articles and observation, that the problem of our habitual misuse of our own bodies has not improved. At least 30 million work days a year in Great Britain are lost through workers in industry having low-back complaints. In large factories with big labour forces, such disorders often pass with less notice than they deserve, but in small units such as shops and farms where physical demands are inescapable and frequently ill-planned, a disability may be seriously disruptive. When back injuries occur, the resulting work-stoppage can be very expensive. The cost to the national economy of sickness through this complaint alone is estimated as in the region of over £87,000,000 per year. If all the other complaints of both men and women were totalled, the national cost would be seen to be tremendous. "The problem is already unmanageably large, certainly too big to be ignored any longer."[22]

Although the scope of physical education has considerably widened during this same period of time and the general health of the school child has improved, the emphasis on different problems has changed.[23] There are still defects of nutrition, for example, as well as an increasing number of obese children. Communicable disease is not now the major problem of school life which it was even twenty years ago. Over the years, the pattern of disease and disability in children has been changing, particularly in the past few decades. Emotional and behavioural disturbances, speech and language disorders, learning difficulties (including those arising from defective vision and hearing), respiratory disorders (particularly asthma), epilepsy and physical handicaps are now the chief disabilities dealt with.

But the fundamental issue of this book, the way children handle themselves, has shown no noticeable change.

There is no intention of usurping the work of the School Medical Service, which now has so many additional problems to deal with. It is agreed that attendance at a remedial centre for treatment to correct some postural fault is very time-consuming and has to be weighed against the loss of education. The solution is rather one of prevention in schools, although children who have already developed unsound habits can also be helped; but the older one becomes the more difficult it is to change a habit. It has been found that children examined in school at eleven years of age have developed faults when examined again at fourteen or fifteen years.

The training of teachers is under serious review; if this approach to education and the learning process is introduced into the training of all teachers during their three- or four-year course nothing but good could result for our children. Teachers wishing to specialise in postural education could take a "wing" course at college, as students do now for other specialist subjects.

Waterloo, it has been said, was won on the playing fields of Eton. Is it not possible that with increased efficiency as the keynote of our national economy and manpower a predominant factor, the economic "battles" of today might well be won in our schools? After all, increased efficiency stems from the sound use of the body and leads to many social and economic advantages. Physical efficiency need not be spartan, mechanical and unemotional. It can mean more freedom, more enjoyment, greater conservation of energy and greater endurance. An attempt to achieve this in school by means of postural education could well improve occupational and industrial efficiency, remove the fundamental cause of many physical and nervous complaints and improve the performance of games and sports.

This approach to physical education can mean as much to the young man planing at his work bench or the young lady pounding her typewriter as to a father digging in his garden or a mother making the beds. It has as much relevance for the junior skipping in the playground as it has for the secondary schoolboy lifting a bar-bell during circuit training. From the infants in the reception class to their grandparents playing bowls the good use of the body will ensure more competent and more comfortable movement and activity.

There is no doubt that the modern conception of posture or management of the body could become an integral part of education today, improving the performance of physical and mental work and preventing many aches and pains later in life.

But skilled use and sound habits must be taught early in life, and here are three possible ways in which adults can help themselves and teachers and parents can help children to learn how to manage themselves effectively. Paradoxically, the first way is by doing nothing positive, merely omitting certain movements or activities, for example, those which contract posture by crushing and compressing the spine, drawing in the joint surfaces and restricting movement and rhythm. Then there is a way of helping children (and ourselves) which is open to the great majority of us: that of helping them to develop sound habits of movement, the correct mechanics, right from the start of school life. By constant repetition these habits could be taught in all school activities or at home in precisely the same way that teachers and parents already try to develop good habits of punctuality, neatness and cleanliness. We could make certain that gross mechanical positions were corrected and that whatever action it performed, the body was used correctly and efficiently. We could encourage children to "ease-up" and to be less tense in classroom activities or at home.

The third way in which help could be given mainly concerns teachers, who could become specialists in postural education, and it is important to remember that such training is not limited to specialists in physical education. Teachers in infant, junior or secondary schools could well become expert in this aspect of education. Indeed, it would be useful if each school had its own specialist in posture in the same way that secondary schools have their special subject teachers. Such a specialist in posture could deal with specific faults individually or in small groups. Normal children would be given attention on the spot, while those who are "physically illiterate" would have special educational treatment (just as retarded readers do) until they showed sufficient improvement to allow them to return to their normal classes.

But whether specialist or not, if each one of us, adult, parent or teacher, could help only one child a term to correct some faulty habit of body management—a million children a year—what a difference this could make to the annual bill of discomfort, pain, lost hours at school or work and money.

"The monetary loss of adults from absence from work can have a number of components. Multiplying the total number of days lost through certified sickness and injury by the average gross remuneration per day of the working population, increased by ten per cent to account for uncertified sickness absence, produces a total figure of £1,750 million for 1967–8. This is of the same order of magnitude as the cost of the National Health Service, some five per cent of National Income."

With these facts in mind it is significant that a 1971 survey comparing causes of incapacity from work between 1954–5 and 1967–8 showed that those causes concerned with management of the body and tension head the list, with very considerable increases in the days lost.[24]

Work days lost from "sprains and strains" *increased* by 267 per cent for males and 131 per cent for females; nervousness and headache by 189 per cent for males and 122 per cent for females; psychoneurosis and psychosis by 152 per cent for males and 302 per cent for females; displacement of intervertebral disc by 147 per cent for males and 113 per cent for females; all injuries and accidents by 72 per cent for males and 46 per cent for females.

There is obviously a rapidly growing problem which must be faced and dealt with. A preventative scheme such as that outlined in this book could do nothing but good; it can be achieved by teaching children how to take such care of their bodies so that they will serve them better, last longer, and actually work and feel at ease; this surely is education for life.

References

1. *Health of the School Child*, H.M.S.O., 1956.
2. Hughes and Hughes, *Learning and Teaching*, Longmans, p. 215.
3. "Postural Abnormalities and their Treatment," *Journal of Physical Education*, 1949.
4. *Journal of Physical Education.*
5. M. E. Todd, *The Thinking Body.*
6. Article in *Future*, Vol. 8, 1953.
7. Dr. W. Barlow, *Nature of Stress Disorder*, pp. 161–4.
8. Dr. W. Barlow, *Nature of Stress Disorder*, pp. 161–4.
9. Wolff, *Headache*, O.U.P., 1958.
10. Dr. W. Barlow, "Anxiety and Muscle-tension Pain," *British Journal of Clinical Practice*, 1959.
11. Dr. W. Barlow, "Anxiety and Muscle-tension Pain," *British Journal of Clinical Practice*, 1959.
12. Dr. W. Barlow, "Anxiety and Muscle-tension Pain," *British Journal of Clinical Practice*, 1959.
13. Dr. W. Barlow, "Anxiety and Muscle-tension Pain," *British Journal of Clinical Practice*, 1959.
14. Dr. W. Barlow, *Nature of Stress Disorder.*
15. Dr. W. Barlow, *Postural Deformity*, 1956.
16. Dr. W. Barlow, *Postural Deformity*, 1956.
17. *The Use of the Self*, Chaterson.
18. Burt, *Proc. Roy. Soc. Med.*, 51. No. 4, 258.
19. Herbert Spencer, *Education.*
20. V. Ogilvie, *Our Times*, Batsford.
21. Dr. W. Barlow, "Anxiety and Muscle-tension Pain," *British Journal of Clinical Practice*, 1959.
22. "Industry and the low-back problem," *New Scientist*, January 1970.
23. *Health of the School Child*, H.M.S.O., 1965.
24. *Off Sick*, Office of Health Economics, 1971.

Glossary

In order to improve the use of one's body it is not necessary to have a detailed knowledge of anatomy and physiology, but some explanation of common terms used in this book may be helpful.

Brachial neuritis: Inflammation, pain and loss of the normal functioning of the muscles in the upper arm.

Cervical spondylosis: Osteo-arthritis of the cervical spine with a locking of the vertebral joint.

Electromygraphic techniques: Methods of measuring the amount of muscular activity during any movement or position held.

Intervertebral discs: These are made of cartilage, and separate the bones of the spine; they are thin button-shaped structures which correspond in shape with the bodies of the vertebrae. These discs are tough, elastic and compressible, varying in thickness in different regions of the spine, being thinnest in the cervical, and thickest in the lumbar, region.

Kyphosis: Sometimes called round back, this is the most common defect, and is invariably accompanied by round shoulders. The head can be the influencing factor; being a relatively heavy part of the body, it can exert considerable leverage on the upper portion of the spine. The further forward it is held, the greater the strain on the muscles of the neck and upper part of the back.

There are many causes of kyphosis which include defective vision and hearing, faulty seating arrangements, poor lighting, overwork and lack of proper exercise, unsuitable clothing, over-rapid growth and debilitating illness. This type of fault usually develops during the years of growth.

Lordosis: Sometimes called hollow back, this is an exaggeration of the curve of the lumbar spine and can lead to an aching in the lower spinal muscles which are held in a constant state of contraction in their effort to maintain the balance of the body. The causes are not so obvious as those which produce kyphosis; the defect is probably due to habit formation during the growing years or to a persistence in some degree of the lordosis which is common in very young children.

Osteo-arthritis: A degenerative disease of the joint leading to pain and deformity and limitation of movement.

Passive spanning exercises: Those where a partner assists the performer and tries to "stretch" the spine in a backward span bend (such movements are now seldom used in physical education programmes).

Psychosomatic disorders: Bodily symptoms produced by psychic, emotional or mental reaction; the whole range of ways in which man interacts with his environment and society, as they relate to the production of illness.

"Refresh": To re-check the postural state after a movement.

Rheumatoid arthritis: Resembling rheumatism, this is a disease affecting the tissues of the joint, which become thickened and inflamed.

Scoliosis: A lateral curving or twisted appearance of the spine (*e.g.* pastry cook, javelin thrower) which may be found in different parts of the vertebral column. Scoliosis may be the first sign of some underlying disease or injury but is often caused through faulty occupational habits, *e.g.* sitting one-sided, or always carrying one-sided.

Spine: The adult spine consists of thirty-three cotton-reel-type bones called vertebrae. During the early months and years of life, in childhood and adolescence, the normal curves of the spine develop and some bones fuse together.

The top seven vertebrae of flattish bones make up the *cervical spine* and form the slight forward curve of the neck region (the knob one can feel at the back of the neck is the seventh cervical); the top two bones are specially adapted to support the skull.

The next twelve vertebrae, which are thicker and more solid make up the *dorsal spine* and form the curve of the shoulders and upper back, with the chest or thoracic region to the front.

The five vertebrae of the lower back, called the *lumbar spine*, are the thickest and strongest in the whole spine, and curve slightly forward.

The bones of the tail end fuse to form the *sacrum* (to which the hip bones are attached) and the *coccyx*, a minute tail that is tucked underneath as we sit.

Static spanning exercises: Arching movements of the spine which are "held" in a position of contraction for a short period of time and then released (again, such exercises are seldom used nowadays).

Trapezii muscles in the neck: These are broad, flat and triangular in shape, lying immediately under the skin of the back. The two muscles together roughly form a trapezium (a four-sided figure with no two sides parallel). These muscles assist in raising, depressing or bracing the shoulders backward and can draw the head backwards (when the shoulders are fixed); acting singly, the muscle can bend the head sideways.